Hypnosis Regression Therapy

*How reliving early experiences
can improve your life*

URSULA MARKHAM

D1421896

PIATKUS

© 1991 Ursula Markham

First published in 1991 by
Judy Piatkus (Publishers) Ltd of
5 Windmill Street, London W1P 1HF

British Library Cataloguing in Publication Data
Markham, Ursula
    Hypnosis regression therapy.
    1. Medicine. Hypnotherapy
    I. Title
    615.8512

ISBN 0-7499-1032-1 (Pbk)

Edited by Esther Jagger
Cover design by Jennie Smith

Photoset in 11/12pt Linotron Baskerville by
Computerset Ltd., Harmondsworth, Middlesex
Printed and bound in Great Britain by
Billing & Sons Ltd., Worcester

*To my mother and father with love and thanks
for giving me such a happy childhood to
look back on*

About the Author

Ursula Markham is a professional hypnotherapist, counsellor and stress management consultant. She is the Principal of the Hypnothink Foundation, and a member of the World Federation of Hypnotherapists and the American Association of Professional Hypnotherapists. She trained in London in 1979 and since 1982 has had her own successful practice in Gloucestershire. She has written several books, and her articles appear in national magazines. She also lectures throughout Britain and has conducted practical workshops for LBC Radio and *Here's Health* magazine as well as for numerous private organisations. Ursula Markham's courses include Self-Hypnosis, Stress Management, Hypnotherapy and Hypnothink Counselling. She has made several audio-cassettes.

'Learning is finding out what you already know.
Doing is demonstrating that you know it.'

Richard Bach, *Illusions*

Contents

Introduction

Not so very long ago, people who consulted a hypnotherapist tended to be seeking help in losing weight,
giving up smoking or overcoming minor habits such as
nail-biting. Today, however, the situation is rather different because the majority of prospective patients are
looking for ways of dealing with deep-rooted problems
which, although they may have a current physical
manifestation, have been caused by an earlier traumatic
emotional experience. Those present-day problems may
range from stammering to fear of relationships; from
phobias to feelings of inadequacy. But one fact is common to all – if the patient is to be helped to eradicate his
problem and to live a full and happy life, he needs to
acknowledge and understand the causes of his present
state. The simplest and most painless way of doing this is
by means of hypnotic regression.

Regression alone is not, of course, the ultimate cure;
indeed it is only the first step on the path. But what an
essential step it is – without it, the treatment itself,
whether by hypnotherapy or any other means, would be
nothing but the superimposing of an artificial veneer of
self-confidence over a troubled inner self. This would
only lead to more problems in the future when the
experiences of the past discovered a new way of invading
the present. It is rather like putting a piece of sticking
plaster over an open wound without first bothering to
clean or treat the wound itself. You might not be able to
see it festering away beneath the dressing, but you can be

sure that it is doing so and that it may even go on to cause more serious – and certainly more painful – problems in the future. In addition, the majority of people find that they have a need to know and understand the reason for their symptoms. Sometimes that need may be on a subconscious level and, if the basic cause were not discovered, the result would be the emergence of a new set of symptoms at a later date.

Every individual has his own subconscious 'filing system' where everything he has ever seen, heard or learnt is permanently stored. Just as with a real filing system, a good deal of what is there is not needed and so it is relegated to the backs of drawers and cupboards to gather dust. Through hypnosis, however, it is possible to search through that filing system in order to find any relevant piece of information the mind may require – although one will be looking at it through different eyes.

Imagine what it would be like if you were suddenly to find a diary which you had kept when you were sixteen years old. The words would describe the feelings and emotions of someone of sixteen, with all the problems, hopes and fears involved. Looking at that diary perhaps twenty years later you would probably smile at how insurmountable some of those problems had seemed to you at the time – and how you wish that they were all you had to worry about today! But that does not mean that, to the sixteen-year-old, those problems were not very real indeed. The effect of those problems upon his life was very real too.

Regression is rather like that. Reliving and re-experiencing a situation through hypnosis is not intended to make you forget past events or pretend that they did not happen. It is just meant to help you to put them in perspective and see that something which may have had a devastating effect on you when you were ten years old (and continued to do so thereafter) has a far less devastating effect when looked at with, say, forty-year-old eyes.

The value of using hypnotic regression in the treatment of a problem – and remember that regression only constitutes one part of the treatment, the ensuing therapy being the other – is that the patient will not get rid of one set of symptoms only to substitute them with another. This is because he has been able to go back and see for himself, hopefully with mature understanding, the original cause of the problem; once he has dealt with that original cause, it no longer needs to have any effect on his present life.

There are two types of regression – (i) to earlier stages in the patient's present life, and (ii) to a possible former life. The actual existence of past lives will be discussed later in this book, but the therapy is equally effective whether one believes that reincarnation is possible or that the facts revealed are simply a product of the patient's subconscious mind.

As will be shown in Chapter 1, hypnosis is not the only available method of inducing regression – but it is the only one I use. Apart from the fact that for many years I have been a practising hypnotherapist, I truly believe that it is the speediest, the most effective and the least painful way of achieving positive results. So it is only regression therapy by means of hypnosis that I shall be discussing in this book. I hope that, by the time you reach the final page, you will be as confident as I am in the technique itself and in its therapeutic value as an improver of lives.

1

The Background to Hypnosis

Hypnosis has been around for a long, long time. No one really knows its origins but it was certainly used therapeutically by the Ancient Egyptians, the Greeks and the Romans. Since that time it has had a somewhat chequered history, at certain times being in favour and at others being disapproved of most heartily. The ancient civilizations were firm believers in a form of hypnosis (although the word itself had not been coined at that time, only coming into existence in the early nineteenth century: it derives from the Greek *hypnos*, meaning sleep). As time went on, however, its curative uses were regarded with more and more suspicion, not assisted by tales such as that of Svengali which helped to convince an already uncertain public that to submit to hypnosis was to give up all free will and to place one's mind in the power of another.

The pioneers of hypnotic regression

It was not until the nineteenth century and the work of Pierre Janet that anyone even began to consider the subject of regression. Janet was a pupil of the well-respected Professor Charcot (1825 – 1893), who was responsible for founding the Salpêtrière School of Hypnotism in France and for bringing credibility to the subject. It was Janet who found, during the course of his work, that patients suffering from what he termed 'neurotic disorders' would often have significant gaps in their

1

long-term memories – they had actually managed to block out incidents from long ago which had been particularly painful or excessively distressing. Using hypnosis, Janet was able to help his patients recall those past events. Such recall led the individual to a deeper understanding of himself and of the traumatic effect on his life of the hitherto 'forgotten' incidents. Understanding, of course, is the essential first step on the path to cure. It is not a painful experience provided the patient is being treated by a trained and ethical therapist who will also give the kind of follow-up treatment described in the case histories detailed in later chapters.

The somewhat better-known Sigmund Freud at one time worked with Janet. It was Freud who made the first extensive use of hypnosis to probe the depths of the subconscious mind. He was also one of the first to insist that the discovery of the root cause of a problem is an essential first stage in the achievement of a cure. Freud's difficulties arose because he did not fully appreciate the need for co-operation between patient and therapist: he was inclined to treat his patients as docile subjects with little or no role to play. Because of this he often failed to bring about cures and eventually became disillusioned with hypnosis as a form of therapy. Today, of course, it is recognized that no real success can be achieved by a therapist working alone; the patient's full co-operation is essential.

Regression gains acceptance

After the time of Pierre Janet and Sigmund Freud, during the first part of the twentieth century, little consideration was given to the subject of regression. Then, as time went on and hypnosis gained credibility and was thought of as more than just a form of stage entertainment, more and more hypnotherapists began to use present-life regression in their work. But the whole concept of past-life regression was thought to be at best

2

unbelievable and at worst as some form of dabbling in an area which would be better left unexplored.

Then came two men who made very significant contributions to the area of past-life regression. One was Morey Bernstein, who worked in the United States, and the other was Arnall Bloxham, who worked in Britain.

Bernstein came into the field of past-life regression almost by accident. As a hypnotherapist, he had been consulted by a lady called Virginia Tighe of Colorado. In the course of treating Mrs Tighe, Bernstein used hypnotic suggestion and then regression, intending to take her back to an earlier time in her current life. But Mrs Tighe claimed that she was able to remember a previous incarnation when she was an Irishwoman by the name of Bridey Murphy. She had never been to Ireland and said that she had never read anything about that country, and yet she was able to supply an abundance of detail about the way of life in that place at an earlier time. All the facts given were checked and were found to be completely accurate. Morey Bernstein was so impressed by this that he published details of the case in a book, *The Search for Bridey Murphy*, in which he gave Virginia Tighe the pseudonym Ruth Simmons.

Many people will have heard of the Bloxham Tapes. Arnall Bloxham was a hypnotherapist working in Cardiff in the sixties and seventies. He was highly respected in his field and became President of the British Society of Hypnotherapists in 1972. Bloxham had always been fascinated by regression to what appeared to be past lives, and he would experiment with those of his patients who proved to be excellent subjects for hypnosis (with their full permission and co-operation, of course), recording the outcome of these experiments. He also held public meetings to discuss the concept of past-life regression, at which he would play to anyone who cared to listen the taped recordings of his experimental sessions. Although his initial interest had been aroused because of the connection between current problems and events which may have taken place in a former life, he became so enthralled by the topic that he took it up for its own sake. In 1976 Jeffrey Iverson published a book about Bloxham and his work called *More Lives Than One?* This book, with a foreword by Magnus Magnusson, became the subject of a BBC television programme at the time.

Today David Canova, Founder and Director of the World Federation of Hypnotherapists, teaches his students, as part of their course, regression (present-life) and re-regression (past-life). In his own practice, if he finds a patient who is a particularly good subject for hypnosis he asks them if they would like to try re-regression for interest's sake; if they agree, with their permission he records the session. Among the more fascinating of his cases is one of a woman (whom I shall call Judith) who, having regressed to being a young woman in a previous lifetime (we'll call her Alice), went on in a later session to regress to being Alice's mother – who, it is interesting to note, had died at the precise moment her daughter was born.

What is hypnosis?

Hypnosis is perhaps the most misunderstood of all the complementary therapies. On the one hand there are those who consider it only one step away from witchcraft, believing that the hypnotherapist is able to subjugate the will and dominate the mind of his unconscious victim. On the other hand, some people see it as instant answer to every problem in life. 'Make me stop smoking,' they cry. 'Make me more confident.' The truth is, of course, that no hypnotherapist can *make* you do anything. His skill lies in helping you to achieve your aim for yourself. Even when you see a stage performance of hypnotism and it seems as though the 'unwilling' subjects are being made to act against their will, that is not really the case. Each of those subjects is, in fact, a willing volunteer and is an extrovert by nature, and so allows himself to become part of the entertainment.

4

Hypnotherapy is a skill which is learnt. It is not, as some people still believe, an almost magical power possessed by just a few. The properly trained hypnotherapist has, like the successful doctor, lawyer or musician, spent a long time studying, practising and perfecting his craft. Because there is no one governing body for hypnotherapists at the time of writing, you will want to ensure that the one you consult has received proper training. Chapter 2 describes some ways of doing this.

CAN EVERYONE BE HYPNOTIZED?

Many people are curious as to who can and who cannot be hypnotized. It is quite simple really. With a few exceptions, anyone who wishes to be hypnotized can be – while anyone who does not wish it cannot. (This applies to the light trance state – see below.)

Anyone who has a history of epilepsy (even if that condition is being fully controlled by medication) should never on any account be hypnotized, as the process of entering the appropriate altered state of mind can actually trigger off an epileptic fit. It might not happen, but it is never worth taking a chance. That, however, is the only case where hypnosis can do harm. In any other situation the worst thing that can occur is that nothing happens at all.

There are really only three types of people who cannot be successfully hypnotized. The first is anyone who is in any way mentally deficient, as such people cannot co-operate sufficiently with the therapist to achieve the desired result. The second is any child under the age of about five, who is unlikely to be able to concentrate for the necessary time – although it must be said that older children probably make the best subjects of all, as they are still at the stage where their imagination is in good working order and they have not become weighed down by the need to earn a living or the problems of bringing up a family. The last category is anyone under the

5

influence of alcohol, as it is well known that the mental faculties of such people are often impaired, even if only temporarily.

So who makes the ideal subject for hypnosis? The best person is someone with the following qualities:

- intelligence
- a good natural memory
- not afraid to express his feelings
- a good visual imagination.

LEVELS OF HYPNOSIS

There are three main levels of hypnosis:

Light trance

There are very few people in whom a light trance cannot be induced should they wish it and provided they are willing to co-operate fully with the therapist.

In this state it is not unusual for the subject to think that he has not been hypnotized at all, but has simply felt very relaxed for a short time. And indeed, this level of hypnosis lies somewhere between the state of deep relaxation and light meditation. It is ideal for those aspects of therapy which do not need to entail regression: giving up smoking, losing weight or training the memory, for example. It is not really suitable for those who need or wish to experience regression. There would probably be some results, but they would probably be somewhat superficial, and the knowledge gleaned would be of a general rather than a specific nature.

Medium trance

This state can be induced in about three-quarters of the population; the rest for some unknown reason cannot achieve it even if they wish to do so. It is, obviously, deeper than the light trance, but not so deep that the patient will not be aware of what is going on around him. He will actually be able to hear any noises which may occur – a telephone ringing or the traffic in the road outside – but those noises are unlikely to impinge on his consciousness or to interrupt his train of thought. They will merely form part of the background.

The medium trance is the best one for any treatment requiring regression, as it will be possible for the patient to relive past experiences on a more realistic level, whether seeing and hearing what takes place or being able to describe it as a spectator.

Deep trance (also known as somnambulistic trance)

This level can only be attained by about 5 – 10 per cent of the population. It is the one most commonly used in stage hypnotism, and the fact that it is beyond the reach of many explains why the stage hypnotist ends up by working with about ten people out of as many as sixty volunteers. By putting those volunteers through a series of rapid tests on-stage, he will soon discover which of them are able of achieving the deep-trance state; it is only these people who will respond quickly and satisfactorily to his suggestions.

I[1] do not believe in using the deep trance state in any form of therapy as it involves hypnoamnesia, a state in which the patient will neither be aware of what is going on at the time nor able to recall it afterwards. I do not consider this ethical in treatment, as I believe that everyone should be fully cognizant of what is happening at each and every stage. Indeed, without such awareness the patient would be unable to co-operate with the therapist and would therefore minimize his chances of a cure. I have never liked any form of 'mystique' in therapy and always take great care to explain to my patients precisely what I am going to do, what I expect of them and what they are likely to experience. (For more details on this, see Chapter 2.) Besides, when talking about therapy by hypnosis – whether the problem requires regression or not – deep trance is never necessary.

---

1. Throughout this book, when I write in the first person singular I am really explaining what any ethical hypnotherapist would do. It is just that it is simpler to write from my own experience.

Even in the deep trance state, no patient will do or say anything which he would not do or say when fully aware and awake. He will not voluntarily do anything which conflicts with his personal moral code, nor can he be induced to do so. The subconscious mind is at all times fully protective and will not allow the patient to betray himself by his actions or his words. Even if he had committed a murder the previous week, he would not betray that fact under hypnosis if he did not wish to!

LEVELS OF ACTIVITY OF THE MIND

Hypnosis takes place in what is called the Alpha state (the subconscious mind). The human mind has four levels of activity:

The Alpha level

This is the level at which we work in hypnotherapy. The Alpha level corresponds to the subconscious and involves almost 100 per cent concentration. You can see, therefore, that when hypnosis is compared to being asleep, nothing could be further from the truth. Neither does it have anything to do with the spontaneous dreams we have when asleep.

The Beta level

This is the level of consciousness at which we all function during our waking hours. Most of this level is involved in the physical functioning of our bodies – breathing, circulation, heartbeat and so on – and no more than a quarter is available for dealing with our conscious thought processes.

The Theta level

This level corresponds to that part of the unconscious mind which functions when we are in a light sleep. In fact, by far the greater part of all sleep takes place on this level.

The Delta level

This is the deep sleep level, at which the unconscious mind is obtaining the greatest amount of real rest. No hypnotic suggestion can be heard when the subject is at the Delta level – which, perhaps surprisingly, occupies no more than about half an hour each night. The actual length of time one is asleep before this level is reached varies from person to person.

FEARS AND ANXIETIES ABOUT HYPNOSIS

Before going any further, perhaps it would be as well to dispel some of the more common myths and fears concerning the subject of hypnosis and to explain my own particular way of working.

As I have said, if a patient does not wish to be hypnotized, then all the skill and expertise in the world will not induce that state in him. Of course, by the time someone comes to see me they have usually made up their mind that hypnosis will be beneficial for them and so this is not a situation I encounter very often. And I always spend the greater part of the first session explaining just what is going to happen and how he is going to feel; as a result I hope that, by the time we begin the hypnosis itself, the patient will have had all his questions answered and his fears allayed, and will have begun to feel confidence in me and what I am about to do.

It is not unusual for someone to wonder whether undergoing hypnosis is likely to induce any unpleasant or harmful side-effects. In all the years I have been practising, and among all the hypnotherapists whom I know or of whom I have read, I have never heard of any individual suffering any side-effects at all – except positive ones. Because the first stage of hypnosis involves learning to relax – something we all need – any side-effects experienced are likely to be very beneficial indeed. You may find that you sleep better than before (and can throw away any sleeping pills you may have been taking), that you have got rid of that nagging headache or that the muscles in your neck and shoulders suddenly feel warm and relaxed.

You can be sure that no harm will ever come to you through hypnosis. Remember that you are always in control, and if there is anything which makes you at all anxious, all you have to do is open your eyes and it is all over. This will do you no harm at all, although to be brought gently back to the present by the voice of the therapist is a more satisfactory way.

When bringing patients out of the hypnotized state I usually count to three. This is done to allow them time to come back gradually to a state of full alertness without any sense of shock – but it would be just as effective if I were to snap my fingers or even simply to tell them to 'wake up'.

Some people also fear that after the session they will be left in a semi-hypnotized state. Or even, as one of my own patients asked me: 'What will happen if you hypnotize me and then drop dead before you wake me up?' Much as I hope this will never occur, all that would happen is that the patient would either open his eyes and come completely out of the hypnotic state, or that he might doze for some ten or fifteen minutes before waking as if from a nap in an armchair.

There are also some patients who make wonderful subjects for hypnotic therapy but who are unable to relax sufficiently for regression. This is normally because they have some fear, conscious or otherwise, about what they will unearth during the course of the treatment. Once again, by the time I have talked to them, explained how regression works and just what they will experience, I would hope that they would feel confident enough in me and in themselves to allow it to take place. And, as I shall explain more fully in Chapter 2, it is quite possible to ensure that they do not suffer in any way at all, whether mentally, physically or emotionally.

Remember that hypnosis is not a party game to be practised by amateurs for the amusement of themselves or others. It is not difficult to learn a simple technique of inducing a hypnotic state in another person – it is knowing how to deal with that person once he is hypnotized which is important, and not to be indulged in for fun. While this would not do any permanent harm to the person being hypnotized, it is not right to treat anyone's problems as subject matter for frivolous experiment.

If hypnosis in any form is to be taken seriously, then it is even more vital that hypnotic regression is treated with due respect. Because the person being regressed may have to face something which was either traumatic at the time or which seemed trivial but has had a long-lasting subconscious effect, the whole subject needs careful and skilful handling. At the end of this book you will find a list of training establishments in hypnosis where students are taught a safe method of regression; they should be able to supply you with the name of an ethical professional hypnotherapist in your area should you require one.

Certain cassette tapes can be bought which are supposed to enable you to experiment with regression yourself. I cannot urge you strongly enough to resist the temptation of trying to work with such tapes. They claim to help you begin a regression by yourself, and then leave you to see where it takes you. All might go well and you might simply relive and re-experience a happy time in your life. The danger arises if you happen to arrive at what was for you a distressing time and there is no one there to help you deal with it in the way I shall describe in Chapter 2.

There is, however, no harm at all in professional hypnotic cassettes, which are designed to assist you in overcoming a specific problem where regression is not needed – smoking, studying, pre-menstrual tension and so on. On these cassettes you will hear the voice of the hypnotherapist, who will help you to achieve the desired state, then give you the same suggestions that he or she would make if you were in the consulting room; finally, the hypnotherapist will wake you up again.

When a patient comes to me for regression, I do in fact record the session on cassette, giving the tape to the patient at the end of the consultation. But these tapes will have blank passages on them, for I never, never record the actual technique. This is not because it is so special or

11

secret that I do not want to divulge it – indeed the patient will remember it quite well for himself – but because I do not want him to listen to that tape at some future date and begin to regress himself when I am not there to take charge of the situation. So the recording will not even begin until the patient has reached that point in his memory which he wishes to explore and, should it be necessary to move him forwards or backwards within that regression, I simply place my hand over the microphone so that the technique is not recorded.

The benefit of self-knowledge

As I pointed out earlier, regression itself does not cure any particular problem. It is merely a first step – but a very significant one, and one without which the hypnotherapist's task would certainly be made far more difficult.

There are some problems (smoking, nail-biting and so on) which can be dealt with without the need for regression. But, apart from the fact that there are some patients who, however straightforward their problem may seem, insist upon knowing what caused it in the first place, self-understanding is the key to the successful resolution of any emotional problem.

This is particularly true when dealing with people who suffer from phobias of one sort or another. The dictionary definition of a phobia is 'an illogical fear', and the sufferer is often quite well aware that his fear is illogical. This fact does nothing to bolster his confidence in himself; without that feeling of confidence, he will find it extremely difficult to work towards overcoming his fear. If regression can find the reason for the initial onset of the phobia – that first, frightening occasion – it may not be sufficient to put an end to it but it certainly stops the sufferer feeling that he is simply being 'weak' and 'foolish' or (as one of my patients put it) that he is 'going out of his mind'. This in turn puts him in the right frame

12

of mind to be helped to overcome the problem once and for all.

So, while regression cannot be claimed to be the be-all and end-all of therapeutic treatment, it is certainly an important stage. To miss it out would make the treatment itself take far longer, if indeed it is to succeed at all.

2

What Happens During Regression Therapy?

Let us suppose you have decided that regression therapy might be helpful to you, either in overcoming a persistent problem or by enabling you to gain further insight into your own spiritual development. Let us also suppose that you have found a hypnotherapist who is both reputable and someone with whom you feel compatible (see p.23). You are bound to have many questions you would like to ask, as well as certain anxieties about which you would like your mind set at rest. Chapters 2 and 3 are designed to help you on both counts. In this chapter I shall set out all those questions which are most frequently asked by prospective patients, and which have not already been covered in Chapter 1; and in Chapter 3, by giving details of the progress of one particular case, I shall endeavour to provide some idea of what to expect during a typical regression therapy session.

It is quite likely that you not only have no experience of regression therapy but have never even been hypnotized before. It is for this reason that a large part of the first consultation is taken up by conversation. The therapist has to take all your details and to ask you certain questions to establish that you are indeed a suitable subject for hypnosis. Then he will go on to tell you about hypnotherapy in general and his own way of working in particular. He will not actually begin treatment of any sort until he is convinced that you are completely comfortable, both with the concept as a whole and with what is going to take place during the particular session.

How will I be hypnotized?

There are various means of inducing hypnosis – but not one of them includes swinging a watch on a chain before your eyes! If you find someone who claims to be a qualified hypnotherapist and who uses this technique, I would advise you to keep looking.

Probably the most common form of induction is by vocal suggestion. This involves the hypnotherapist talking you gently and quietly through a basic relaxation exercise which is not unlike the early stages of yoga. This should include establishing a regular pattern of breathing which will, of course, make that relaxation even deeper.

In most cases you will be asked to close your eyes so that you will not be distracted by your surroundings. Sometimes pleasant mental images will be suggested – perhaps a walk in a country lane or along a seashore. Some therapists like to have gentle meditative music playing in the background, while others prefer absolute stillness. The induction will also include the suggestion that your limbs are growing increasingly heavy, although your mind will always be clear and you will be completely aware of all that is happening. This part of the session will continue until the therapist is certain that you have fully entered the hypnotic state.

It is also possible to induce hypnosis by means of fascination. This can take more than one form. You may be asked to concentrate on a pinpoint of light or on a particular spot on the ceiling while the therapist makes his suggestions of relaxation. This helps your eyes to grow tired and your eyelids heavy, so that you soon feel you need to close them.

Another form of fascination is to concentrate on the hypnotic spiral, which is a large disc bearing black lines which disappear to a single central point. This has a similar effect and you will begin to grow drowsy and relaxed as the hypnotherapist speaks to you.

What will it feel like?

You will feel very relaxed and comfortable. Perhaps the easiest way to explain is to ask you to imagine what it feels like to be lying tucked up, snug and warm, in your own bed at night and being somewhere in that half-and-half land where you are neither completely asleep nor fully awake.

If someone very close (a member of your family, for instance) were to come into the room while you were in that state, you would be aware of it but you probably would not move or do anything about it because it felt 'right'. If, however, an unwelcome intruder were to enter the room, you would be instantly wide awake. Hypnosis is rather like the former situation; you are aware of all that is happening but, because it feels so right and so pleasant, you allow it to happen.

Your mind will be in complete control throughout the session. You will not be unconscious at all, but will be able to hear and understand every word that is said. After all, if you are being asked to co-operate with the hypnotherapist, it is important that you should be aware of what is going on. Also, it is vital from the point of view of ethics that you can hear and understand what is going on. Because you are so aware, you may even hear background noises outside, and you will certainly hear the therapist's voice. None of these things, however, should intrude upon your relaxed and pleasant state.

Should I wear anything special?

As long as you are comfortable, there are no hard and fast rules about clothing. But comfort is vital – so avoid very tight waistbands, very high collars or shoes which pinch. Indeed, many people prefer to remove their shoes when being hypnotized, as they find this more comfortable. It is also advisable not to wear contact lenses, as you will have your eyes closed for quite a long time, usually about twenty minutes.

Is it all right to eat or drink before a session?

Because hypnosis is concerned with your sense of well-being, and the more comfortable you are the more you will be able to relax, it is wiser not to consume a huge meal immediately beforehand. Equally it would be foolish to have starved yourself so that you were hungry enough to feel discomfort. You need to be concentrating on the hypnosis rather than on the emptiness or heaviness of your stomach!

I prefer my patients not to have had alcoholic drinks just before a session. You would be surprised to know how little alcohol is needed to affect your concentration; you certainly do not have to be drunk. If you have had more than a little alcohol you would probably become so relaxed that you fell asleep and nothing the therapist was saying would register at all. You would be wasting not only the therapist's time but your own money too.

So use your common sense. A light meal without alcohol about an hour or so before your treatment is just about right.

What will I have to do?

All you have to do is to be willing to co-operate with the hypnotherapist as he gently takes you through the relaxation exercise to the hypnotic state. You will either be lying on a couch or sitting in a comfortable chair with a back high enough to support your head. You will not normally be asked to speak during this induction period. Indeed, many forms of treatment by hypnosis do not call for the patient to utter a word. Naturally, this is not so in the case of regression therapy. But certainly during these early stages the most you will usually be asked to do is to nod your head or say 'yes' at appropriate times.

Suppose I am taking prescribed medication?

With the exception of epileptics (see p.5) – even those whose condition is being kept well under control by prescribed drugs – there is no way that any other form of medical treatment or medication can affect your ability to be a good hypnotic subject. It works the other way around too; hypnotic therapy cannot have any adverse effect upon whatever form of medical assistance you might be receiving.

What if I have a poor visual imagination?

The use of the imagination is one of the vital components of successful hypnotherapy, whether regression is involved or not. Your imagination is possibly one of the greatest gifts you possess and it is up to you to cherish and improve it.

Although many people have been known to claim that they have a poor visual imagination, this is not in fact so. Like any other part of the body it may have become weak through disuse, but it is a fact that the only people who do not have the ability to 'see' clearly in their minds are those who were born blind. Anyone who can see – or who has ever been able to see – is able to visualize. If you feel that your powers of visualization are not as strong as they might be, there is a simple series of exercises you can practise in order to improve them.

1. Choose a simple, everyday object (perhaps a vase, a jug or a lamp). Study that object for several minutes. Don't just look at it and think to yourself 'That's a jug' and leave it at that. Look at it in detail. Be aware of its shape, its colour, how the handle fits on to it and so on. Now close your eyes and try to visualize that object in your mind, seeing it in precisely the same detail as before. If you find it difficult, simply open your eyes and take another look at it before closing them again and repeating the process.

2. Once you find that you can visualize a single item, repeat the process with a group of three or four. Look at them closely before closing your eyes and trying to see them in your mind.

3. Now you need to experiment with a more abstract image. Think of a place that you remember from your recent or distant past. It is not necessary to remember the specific events which occured there – although there is no harm in doing so – but try to recreate that place in your imagination in the greatest detail possible. Once you can do this successfully, you can never again claim that you have a poor visual imagination.

Don't expect to rush through this routine overnight. Just as a weak muscle needs repeated exercise, so too does a weak imagination. But both can be greatly improved with regular practice.

Do I need to do anything between visits?

When treating a patient without the use of regression, I always send him away with 'homework' to do. This does not mean that they will have to hypnotize themselves, although some people are in fact taught self-hypnosis. They will simply be asked to spend about fifteen minutes a day using a combination of relaxation and visualization techniques which they will have been taught.

The work that a patient does on himself between visits is just as important as the work we do together during the consultations. For one thing, the repetition helps to reinforce whatever suggestion he may have been given; and, for another, I consider it vital that the patient realizes he is playing an extremely significant part in his own cure. This belief not only increases the beneficial effects of the specific therapy but also helps him to become more confident in general as well as in his ability to change anything about himself or his life that he does not like.

The best time for this 'homework' to be done is in what I call the twilight time at night – that period when he is in bed and drowsy but not yet asleep. I have known patients to be worried because they have on occasion fallen asleep while practising – but in fact this does not matter. The instructions about practising will have been given while he was under hypnosis (although he will, of course, have heard and understood every word) and so, because he is willing for it to happen, they will be firmly planted in his subconscious mind.

Now when you go to sleep it is only the conscious mind which shuts down; the subconscious cannot do so. So whatever suggestion is in the subconscious will continue to have effect even if the patient is not sufficiently alert to notice it. It is rather like someone switching on a cassette in one room and then walking into another. The cassette will continue to play, whether he is there to listen to it or not.

THE REGRESSION SESSION

The situation is slightly different where regression is concerned. The regression session will often take place during the first or second consultation, and no home-work as such will follow this. The regression alone will probably have raised enough points for the patient to consider during the ensuing period without him having any other work to do. In fact, I usually like to leave a full two weeks between the regression and the continuation of treatment. This is partly because the memories un-covered may well trigger off others quite spontaneously, and also because the patient will need time to mull over the situation at his leisure. Once the actual follow-on treatment begins, however, he will definitely be asked to do some work on his own at home.

If I feel that a particular patient is suffering from extreme tension and finds it difficult to relax, then I may suggest that, during the two weeks following the regres-sion session, he simply practises a basic relaxation exercise for a few minutes a day. This will be of great help to both of us when we come to continue his therapeutic treatment.

How long will each consultation last?

It is very hard to give a precise answer to this question as, to a certain extent, it will vary from person to person. But, as a general guideline, the initial consultation (the one which includes the regression itself) will probably take about one hour. Of that hour, about half of the time will be spent taking notes of the patient's problem and explaining about hypnosis in general and regression in particular. If the outcome is to be successful, it is vital that all anxieties and fears are dealt with before treatment is begun.

The regression itself will last approximately twenty minutes – the maximum length of time the human mind is able to concentrate sufficiently to allow it to take place. The final ten minutes or so of the session will be spent discussing what has arisen, how the patient feels about it, and the way future treatment is likely to proceed.

If follow-up therapy is to ensue, those consultations are likely to take a little less time – anything from thirty to fifty minutes. During this time the patient will report on what has occurred since the last meeting and we will discuss what is to happen during the current visit. Once again the period of hypnosis itself will take only about twenty minutes, after which we will decide what the best form of homework would be in the particular circumstances.

How do I find a good hypnotherapist?

Unfortunately no single governing body for hypnosis exists at the time of writing. Here, instead are some helpful hints:

1. Write to one of the reputable training establishments for a list of practitioners in your particular area. You will find several of these establishments listed on p.121. I have chosen to give details only of those of whose standards and courses I have personal knowledge, but I

would emphasize that there may also be other places which are also of a very high standard. In addition, there are some excellent hypnotherapists who just do not have the right personality to work in the field of past-life regression – and, of course, there are others who simply do not wish to. So do ask lots of questions to make sure that the hypnotherapist you choose is right for the kind of treatment you want.

2. Never be afraid to ask your chosen hypnotherapist about his training and qualifications.

3. Any reputable hypnotherapist should be quite prepared to have a ten-minute 'chat' with you, free of charge, during which he can answer any questions you might have. Naturally you should not expect this to be a full consultation, but it should give you time to see how you relate to the particular therapist concerned and how much confidence you feel in him.

4. It is also important to find a hypnotherapist who is prepared to be frank and open with you and to answer all your questions. Beware of the therapist who is so anxious to preserve the myth of 'special power' that he is not willing to tell you everything you wish to know. Hypnotherapy is not a God-given gift but a skill which is learnt – although some people have more of an aptitude for it than others. There should never be any mystique involved in a course of hypnosis, whether regression is part of the treatment or not.

5. I would advise against choosing a hypnotherapist who is anxious from the outset to charge you for a complete course of treatment. No one can know precisely how many consultations are involved in treating a specific individual. Naturally experience enables one to give a reasonable estimate – but we are constantly being taken by surprise, both by those who manage to overcome their problems amazingly quickly and by others who take longer than was initially estimated. Because of this I believe it is unethical to charge for, say, ten consultations when it may well turn out that only six are necessary.

I do, however, feel that any therapist is justified in asking you each time to pay in advance for your next visit (which would result in no payment on the day of the final consultation). In this way, should you be unable to attend at the last moment and he has to sit twiddling his thumbs in his consulting room because it is too late to give the appointment to anyone else, he is recompensed for the wasted time.

6. Listen to what others tell you. There is no form of advertising so valuable as word of mouth. If a friend or colleague whose opinions you respect tells you that he or she has received beneficial treatment from a particular hypnotherapist, perhaps that is the one for you to consult.

7. Perhaps the most important piece of advice of all is to trust your own instincts. If you take an instant dislike to a particular hypnotherapist, or if you feel that you are unlikely to be able to establish any rapport with him, then he is not the one for you and any treatment would be unlikely to succeed. This need not mean that he is no good at his job – simply that he is not the right person to help you. Because all therapists realize that this can be the case, no one is likely to be offended if you feel that you would prefer to consult someone else.

Can I learn to be a hypnotherapist?

The ability to treat others by means of hypnosis is an acquired skill and not a special gift possessed by only a few. Of course it is necessary for the prospective student to possess a reasonable amount of intelligence as well as a genuine desire to help others. While it is not difficult to learn the techniques necessary to enable you to hypnotize other people, the real test of skill and acquired knowledge comes in knowing how to help them deal with their problems once you have done so.

Any of the training establishments listed in the back of this book will be happy to send you details of their own courses in hypnotherapy.

All the questions so far have related to hypnotherapy in general – whether or not regression forms part of that treatment. Because in recent years hypnosis has tended to leave behind its mystical and Svengali-related image – and also because complementary medicine in general is far more widely accepted than it used to be – many people are less worried about the whole concept than before.

The same cannot yet be said about the idea of regression. A great deal of the blame must be laid at the feet of those who link regression with occult activities or treat it as some sort of parlour-trick to be practised for fun at parties. It is therefore understandable that, even among those who now happily accept the idea of hypnotherapy, there is still a certain amount of reservation about the concept of regression as part of the healing process. It is for this reason that so much of the initial consultation is spent explaining the technique to the patient, answering all his questions and, hopefully, dissolving all his apprehensions. These are the questions that are typically asked during that initial consultation:

Why and when is regression more beneficial than simple hypnotherapy?

When an individual is faced with a situation or an event which is highly traumatic, his instinctive reaction is often to block it from his memory. Sometimes this is done quite deliberately – he refuses to think about the event at all – while at other times it is his subconscious mind which ensures that he is no longer troubled by it. In many cases treatment is enhanced, as well as accelerated, when such memories are recalled. Often the individual has done such a good job of 'forgetting' that this recall can only be achieved by means of regression.

Regression therapy does not play a role in all hypnotic treatment: if the patient wishes to give up smoking or to pass his driving test, for instance, then regression does not come into it. The real value of regression therapy is demonstrated when the patient is aware of how he or she acts in certain circumstances but can find no reason for it at all. It is only by means of regression that the root of such cases can be discovered and the foundation laid for the follow-up treatment. In addition, for those involved on a journey of spiritual exploration and discovery, a series of regressions is of great benefit as it brings to light the pattern so far and allows the patient to make decisions about how he intends to progress.

How many sessions of regression will I need?

I am afraid that this is rather like asking 'How long is a piece of string?' as there is no hard and fast answer.

For someone who is having regression therapy to uncover a traumatic event earlier in this present lifetime, a single session may well suffice. There are two main reasons for this. First of all, the person concerned is already thinking about the problem and how to overcome it, so the subconscious mind is already working on the situation, whether one is aware of it or not. Secondly, the experienced hypnotherapist will know how to take the patient back in time, beginning with a relatively happy time of life before progressing to the period where the trauma occurred. In this way the patient's confidence grows during the course of the single session and he is able to bring to the forefront of his mind the relevant period in his life.

If you are having regression therapy to help you deal with a problem whose roots are buried in a previous existence, you may well need two or three sessions of actual regression before you hit upon the significant lifetime. Remember, the protectiveness of your subconscious is unlikely to allow you to go straight to a period or an event so traumatic that it has affected you for such a long time afterwards. There are exceptions to this rule, of course. Patients who have had previous experience of hypnotherapy (even if no regression was involved) are more likely to have confidence in the technique and in its safety, and therefore are often more willing to put themselves in the hands of the therapist and trust their own subconscious.

For those who wish to learn more about their spiritual evolution and development through the technique of regression, there will naturally be a number of sessions involved in establishing a pattern which can be clearly seen. However, in such cases one will often not need to progress to the follow-up sessions of therapy which would be needed by those others who are trying to overcome a particular problem.

How will I be regressed?

I do not intend to give the precise wording of a regression session on these pages because some readers might try to use it in the wrong way.

What I will say in answer to the question is that I personally always use hypnosis as the first stage of any regression session. This ensures that the patient's conscious mind is sufficiently relaxed to allow the subconscious to offer up whatever it may choose to reveal. Because the hypnotherapist is present the whole time and observing the patient's reactions, it is also possible for him to know when to introduce the detachment technique which will ensure that no distress is suffered.

What is this detachment technique?

Imagine that you are watching a home movie of yourself as a small child of seven or eight years old. In that film you see yourself falling over, grazing your knees quite badly and, not surprisingly, crying. The adult you – the one watching the film – would know perfectly well that the fall had hurt and distressed you and would be able to

26

say so. But your knees would not actually hurt *now*. You could feel sympathy for the child that you were, but you would not actually experience that pain today.

By using the detachment technique during the course of the regression, it is possible for the hypnotherapist to ensure that you do not suffer in any way – if, for example, you are undergoing past-life regression and you came to a painful and untimely end in an earlier life. After all, if you had been hanged, drawn and quartered at a time when such deaths were not uncommon, you would not really want to feel either the physical pain or indeed the terror which must have accompanied it!

I do not agree with certain therapists who insist that, unless an experience is relived with all the accompanying trauma, no benefit is gained. It is quite sufficient to *know* and understand what happened – there is absolutely no need to suffer, whether physically, mentally or emotionally. In fact, I would not be able to conduct sessions of regression therapy – whether present- or past-life – if I thought that my patient was going to go through agonies while it was going on.

This is another reason for believing that the best regressions take place under hypnosis. Due to the protection of that ever-watchful subconscious mind, a hypnotic subject will show early signs of approaching stress; so it is possible for the hypnotherapist to take avoiding action and to put the detachment technique into practice. As soon as I see that a patient's breathing pattern is changing dramatically or that the eye movement behind the closed lids is altering, I instruct him to be aware of and to understand all that is happening but to see it as if on a film or television screen, so that he is completely detached and feels no physical or mental distress whatsoever. And because this technique will have been explained to him during the early part of the consultation, he will find it quite simple to do.

How will I know whether I have been regressed or whether it is simply my imagination working overtime?

In the case of regression to earlier times in your present life, there will be enough evidence for you to check on at a later date, even if you are not actually aware of specific people or events. Even if no one is around who can confirm a particular incident, if you are able to come up with details of surroundings and personalities of which you had no conscious memory, and if these are later proved to have been accurate, there is no real reason to suppose that a significant event was simply a figment of an over-active imagination.

The question takes on a different quality, however, when related to regression to what was possibly a former life (see Chapter 6). How will you know whether it is genuine regression or something you have imagined? In many cases you will not be sure – particularly if this is your first experience of regression therapy.

Some people, after an experience of regression to a past life, are absolutely convinced in their own minds that it was a genuine recollection of a time when they have lived before. Others are not so sure. Once again I would ask – does it really matter? Since the object of the session in the first place was to play a part in helping the patient to deal successfully with a problem which has been troubling him, provided the session fulfills that role we do not need to worry unduly about whether it was a real regression experience or not (although, as I have already stated, I feel quite strongly that the majority of cases are indeed genuine). If it was a product of the patient's imagination, there would have to be a very significant reason why the subconscious mind should choose to create a particular series of events and personalities.

The one thing I do ask all my patients is that they try not to question whether or not the regression is real during the course of the session itself. i am certainly in favour of questioning, both on my part and that of the

28

patient, but it is better to do this towards the end of the consultation when the regression itself is over. The reason for this is that the more spontaneous the answers given during the session, the more worthwhile they are likely to prove. If the patient hesitates before each answer, wondering whether or not his imagination has come into play, he will be quite unable to be spontaneous and will in fact break the train of the regression completely, often bringing the session to an end. Since he will afterwards have a perfectly clear memory of all that has occurred – plus, of course, the whole thing recorded on cassette – there will be plenty of time for questioning the genuineness of the regression at his leisure.

Will I know what is going on?

Yes, at all times you will hear and understand every word. In fact, I consider this vital as far as the therapeutic value of the treatment is concerned. It is important to be able to think about what has taken place once the session is over and to know that all the things you said were a product of your own subconscious and therefore likely to be extremely relevant to your own development.

It is quite difficult to explain to someone who has not experienced past-life regression how they will feel. At no time will you lose track of your present persona; that will remain with you, even if it is somewhat in the background. However, you will at the same time be aware that you are 'someone else' with different feelings, emotions and experiences. It is because you do not lose touch with your present identity that I hesitate to ask the question 'What is your name?' too early in the session; the patient's instinct would be to answer by giving me today's name. I prefer to build up an image of character, personality and surroundings before establishing such details as name, date and so on.

You will, in fact, be so much in control of the situation that, should you decide at any moment that you do not wish to continue, all you have to do is open your eyes and you will be your present-day self again, exactly as you were when you first entered the consulting room.

Will I see pictures in my mind?

People vary greatly and may well experience regression in many different ways. Some will actually feel that they are inside the body of the former self, and that everything is going on around them just as it does in ordinary life. Others will talk about themselves as 'he' or 'she' and describe what is taking place as though it were happening to a character in a television play. Some people *see* very clearly and are able to describe actual images; others do not actually see anything at all but *know* what is going on and are able to relate to it. This does not make the experience any less valid; it is simply an indication of the difference between the visual powers of one person and another. 'Knowing' is just as accurate as 'seeing'. After all, you do not have to look at your feet to know what shoes you have on.

How do you build up the picture in a regression session?

When dealing with regression to an earlier stage in this lifetime, I like to try and go back initially to a relatively happy time in the patient's life. Often I ask him to remember a birthday, an outing or a holiday, and we start to build the image from there. In some cases, where the childhood has been unhappy or deprived, there is no such happy occasion to build upon; in such instances I start by asking the patient to tell me what he could see as he lay in bed at night – this often brings its own feelings of security to even the unhappiest child.

If we are dealing with a regression to what may be a former lifetime, then, having asked the patient to go back to a period with which his subconscious mind feels comfortable, I like to help him to create the picture of his former personality little by little. Perhaps I will begin by asking him to tell me what he is wearing, what his hair is like, whether his skin seems to be that of someone who is young or of an older person. I might then ask him to look at his hands and see whether they are those of someone who does manual work or whether they seem to belong to a well-to-do person. Gradually I will extend the picture to take in the surroundings: town or country, soft grass or cobbled path, warm sunny day or frost and snow . . . and so on. It actually takes some time before I get to the stage of asking for his name, the date or details of the place where he lives.

By building the picture up slowly in this way, the patient is not suddenly confronted with demands for details before he has settled comfortably into the personality and environment of the person he once was. Such confrontation could so interrupt the subconscious flow that he would, in fact, be brought back with a jolt to the present time and would be unable to continue with the regression at all.

Will I always have been the same sex?

In previous lives we have been both male and female, both bad and good. It is generally accepted that each person, man and woman, is made up of both masculine and feminine qualities, and it appears that in some lifetimes the masculine will have been predominant while in others it will have been the feminine. And, if one accepts the concept that the spirit is journeying through many lifetimes in order to achieve that degree of evolution which makes it unnecessary to spend further time on this earth, then surely it must be essential to experience life both as a man and as a woman.

This question indicates one of the reasons why I ask patients to answer questions as spontaneously as possible.

Otherwise a very 'macho' man might feel embarrassed at having to say that he feels he is living as a fragile teenage girl.

Does one experience past lives in reverse chronological order?

No, the order seems to be fairly haphazard – and I feel that this is to the benefit of the patient. Remember that regression is a new experience for your subconscious mind and it will do whatever is necessary to protect you. Suppose, for example, that your most recent life had been a particularly horrifying and traumatic one: you would not really want to experience it the first time you were regressed, as you might not be able to cope. Once you have experienced regression a couple of times, however, you will have grown more confident in the technique, in the fact that the therapist is able to ensure that you come to no harm and in your own control of the situation. In such circumstances and, with the aid of the detachment technique (see p.26) you will be able to cope with any situation which may arise.

The first time you experience a previous life, you will probably find that the life itself was relatively uneventful. You will have lived your lifetime and finally died having experienced nothing more traumatic than the normal ups and downs that any individual has to encounter. Of course, the fact that you discover that you have lived before at all is exciting in itself, particularly if you are able to remember details which can later be corroborated.

To me, the fact that most lives are relatively uneventful is more convincing than if we were all able to give details of thrilling and unusual events or lives of fame and fortune. After all, at any one time in man's history, there are far more 'ordinary' people (and I do not mean that in a derogatory sense) than those who hit the headlines.

In past-life regression, will I progress from childhood to adulthood?

Not necessarily. Because I do not want to influence the mind of the patient in any way, the phrase I usually employ is: 'Go to wherever your subconscious mind feels comfortable.' Now this may mean being a person of six years old or sixteen or sixty. Whichever point the patient selects, that is the age from which I start to build up a picture of the character. Then, if it seems necessary, it is possible to go either backwards or forwards in time *during that same lifetime* to complete the picture.

Will I know anyone in my former life whom I know in my present one?

Once again I can only speak from my own experience of what my patients have told me.

It appears that one progresses from life to life with the same nucleus of people around one – although casual acquaintances on the outer edge may change. Relationships may vary; the mother in one lifetime may be the companion in another. The grandson of today may have been the beloved teacher of centuries ago. It is interesting to note that, even when the person concerned has changed age, appearance and even sex, the patient undergoing the regression is none the less perfectly aware of who they are.

You will know that, in your present life, you can meet someone new and within no time at all that person becomes a true friend. You may have known someone else for twenty years and yet he will never be more than a casual acquaintance. Could it be that the friend is actually someone whom you recognize from a previous life, and that is why you immediately feel that you have a mutual link?

Do you ever cover more than one previous life in a single session?

I cannot speak for other hypnotherapists, but for myself I do not think it is a good idea. It is not simply the information brought to the fore during the session itself which is significant, but also anything which may come to the patient's mind between the end of that consultation and the beginning of the next. This might happen because he chooses to listen to the recording of the regression, or it might arise spontaneously. In either event, I believe that it could only cause confusion if we were dealing with more than one previous life at a time.

I have aimed to answer all the questions usually asked (and a few more besides), but do remember that, whichever hypnotherapist you consult, he or she should be quite willing to do precisely the same for you and to put your mind at rest about anything else which may be troubling you with regard to regression therapy as well as to hypnosis itself.

3

A Typical Case Study

I would like to take you, stage by stage, through a typical case so that you may know precisely what to expect in both present-life and past-life regression. The patient, whom I shall call Maxine, first came to see me because she had a phobia about water – a phobia which was becoming so exaggerated that she could not even bear to put her hands in water and had to rely on creams and lotions to cleanse her face and body.

The first thing Maxine said to me when she entered my consulting room was that she hoped she was not wasting my time and she was sorry she was being so stupid. She sat in the chair looking down at her hands, at the floor – anywhere but at me. Her voice was little more than a whisper. She told me that she did not quite know where to begin.

I did my best to reassure her that I would not think her stupid, no matter what her problem. Indeed, it takes quite a wise person to be sufficiently aware that they have a problem to seek professional help.

The basic problem

Slowly and painfully the story came out. Ever since she was a little girl Maxine had been terrified of water. She certainly had not been able to learn to swim when the other children did; in fact she had constantly been in trouble at school because she would invent any excuse to avoid even going near the swimming pool. On the few occasions when she had been compelled to enter the water, she had stayed in the very shallowest part of the pool and had never for a moment released her grip on the handrail.

Initially the problem seemed to apply only to such expanses of water as swimming pools, rivers and the sea. Not for Maxine the fun of a seaside holiday. She would play happily on the sand for hours as long as the tide was out but would run from the beach as soon as the sea came to within several yards of where she was sitting.

Matters get worse

Had the problem remained static, Maxine might never have come to see me. After all, although it can be inconvenient if one is frightened of swimming pools or beaches, they are both situations which can be avoided. But gradually her horror of water had extended to the bath and shower in her own home. By the time she was ten years old the nearest she came to having a bath was to stand on the bathmat and sponge herself down. Her parents, although they loved their daughter, were not the most understanding of people and assumed that she was being disobedient. Her older brother and sister found out about the situation and teased her unmercifully. From being a relatively happy, if somewhat timid, little girl Maxine became shy and secretive and spent many hours playing alone, either in the garden or in her bedroom.

As she grew older the problem took on mammoth proportions. By covering her hands and lower arms in the most enormous pair of rubber gloves she could just about force herself to help with the washing up. But washing her hair was such torture that she eventually decided that, whatever the expense, she would pay a weekly visit to a hairdresser. In this way, although she hated the feeling of water on her head, she did not have to become involved in the actual washing process herself.

The decision to seek professional help

Then came the moment when she finally realized that she needed professional help. For some time she had done all that was possible to avoid going out in the rain as she could not bear the thought of the water touching her skin. She had not been able to hold down a job because of her phobia – no one is really willing to employ someone who will only come into the office on fine days, particularly in England! Fortunately her husband was in a good position financially, and so any money she might have earned was not essential to boost the family budget. But one fine day in early summer when the sky was blue and there was not a cloud in the sky, Maxine found herself cancelling an arrangement to meet a friend in town. She made some weak excuse when she telephoned to break the appointment, but she knew perfectly well that she was apprehensive about going out *in case* the weather changed and it began to rain. Suddenly she realized that her phobia was beginning to make her a prisoner in her own home, and that it was about time she sought help in overcoming it.

Initial fears and doubts

During the first consultation a great deal of time was taken up listening to Maxine's story and reassuring her that her problem was not incapable of being solved, although at that stage I was not quite certain how long this would take. Poor Maxine had such a low opinion of herself that it was going to be necessary to build up her confidence in general, so that she would then be able to play a part in her own treatment.

So doubtful was Maxine about her ability to contribute to the treatment in general, and about the strength of her visual imagination in particular, that we decided between us to do no more than practise relaxation and visualization techniques during that first visit. After a couple of false starts, Maxine was actually able to relax relatively well and she found that she had no problems about imagining a pleasant scene in her mind provided the visualization was guided by me. She was absolutely terrified of creating her own image in case she found that some expanse of water found its way into the picture. For this reason I made a cassette of the particular imagery I used and asked Maxine to practise using it (in combination with the relaxation technique) for a week before coming to see me again.

The decision to use regression

By the second visit Maxine had become quite adept at using the techniques I had taught her. Indeed, she told me that she looked forward to practising them each evening as it formed such a peaceful interlude in her anxious life. I had already come to the conclusion that regression therapy would probably be the best way to help Maxine, and I put the idea to her. This was something she had never even heard of, so we spent quite a long time discussing hypnosis, regression and how the techniques could be applied to her situation. Maxine asked me a number of the usual questions, and I answered each one in turn hoping to set her mind at rest. Eventually she agreed with me that no harm could come from using regression therapy, particularly when I assured her that, should she change her mind at any point, all she had to do was open her eyes and the session would automatically come to an end.

The rejection of present-life regression

We first discussed the possibility of regressing to a very early period in her current life. However, Maxine informed me that her mother had always described how she had screamed when being bathed as a tiny baby, so she doubted whether we would be able to find a specific incident which could have caused the onset of the phobia. Although it is actually possible to regress a patient to babyhood and even to the mother's womb, I felt that perhaps in Maxine's case we should try past-life regression (see Chapter 6).

Past-life regression: the first session

Although I had already spoken to her about past lives, Maxine was not at all sure that she believed in the concept. I explained that this would make no difference as the results would be the same, whether the past lives were real or simply figments of her imagination. After all, if the images were created by her subconscious mind, there must be a reason why it chose to create certain images and not others. Reminding her that she would still be in full control at all times, I asked her whether it was not worth trying the technique to see what happened. I also told her that there was no guarantee that she would come up with the answer the first time she was regressed, as this would be a new experience for her and her ever-protective subconscious would not want her to be upset in any way.

Armed with these reassurances, Maxine decided to try past-life regression and see what happened. Despite her earlier fears, she proved to be an excellent subject, probably due in part to her desperation to be helped and partly to the fact that she had spent a week practising the relaxation technique and listening to my voice on cassette, so that she was comfortable with both.

As I questioned her during the session, Maxine described to me a life as Martha, a fisherman's wife in a small seaport in the late eighteenth century. She was able to describe in minute detail her clothes, her home and even what the fishing boats and the harbour were like. It was a fairly uneventful life, seeming to begin and end in that one small harbour town. Nothing traumatic happened; there were just the ordinary ups and downs which would naturally have occurred in the life of a humble family striving to make a reasonable living in a somewhat precarious way. I found it interesting, however, that Maxine – or Martha – experienced no anxiety due to the nearness of the sea, even when she described to me a violent storm when giant waves lashed the walls of the seaside dwellings. She simply told me how relieved she was that her husband had not put to sea that day.

At the end of the session, I brought Maxine back to the present time and out of the hypnotic state and asked her what she felt. She had been so engrossed in Martha's life that it had not even crossed her mind that she (Maxine) should be frightened of that great expanse of water. Of one thing she was convinced, however, and that was that she had actually regressed to a previous life and that it had not simply been the work of her imagination. This is a very common occurrence when someone who is a good subject experiences past-life regression, although they – and, indeed, I – find it difficult to explain just how they *know* the regression was real. Maxine told me that she had known all the time that she was her twentieth-century self and that she was sitting in a comfortable chair in my consulting room. Yet at the same time she knew that she actually was Martha – she felt like Martha deep within her and had, in fact, completely forgotten *why* she was being hypnotized and regressed. Although that session had not given any indication of why her water phobia had begun, at least it had shown her that there was a time before it existed. She was not only confident that a future session would reveal its origins, she was anxious to try again as soon as possible.

The second session

A week later Maxine arrived for her next consultation. So eager was she to experience another session of past-life regression that she was fifteen minutes early for her appointment! I explained to her that, although I could make no promises, since she now felt much more confident about the technique it was quite possible that this session would reveal the cause of her phobia.

As she was now used to the technique, Maxine slipped quickly and easily into the regression. This time she told me that she was a lad called Daniel, the younger son of a schoolteacher and his wife in a small town in the south of England. Initially she went right back to the age of four and, although she could not tell me what year it was, she did know that there was a queen called Victoria.

One day in the summer, young Daniel had gone for a walk along the towpath of a nearby canal with his older brother and two or three other 'big boys'. Quite how it happened he was not sure, but at some point he had slipped and fallen into the canal. Being unable to swim, he had gone under water several times before being rescued and carried to safety by Richard, his brother. Although he was naturally distressed, this mishap did not seem to have any permanent effect upon him. In fact he was so attracted to the canal with its brightly painted barges pulled by strong horses that his parents finally had to forbid him to go there in case he had another accident. Of course, one of the effects of these repeated cautions was to link the idea of 'accident' and 'water' in the young boy's mind.

The matter might well have ended there, with no long-term ill effects for Maxine, were it not for the fact that poor Daniel was to have another unfortunate experience with the canal.

Some years passed. Daniel was now sixteen and working as clerk to a lawyer in the town. Walking home from his job one payday, he was set upon by two young men who hit him with a stick, pushed him to the ground and seized his meagre wages. Daniel struggled but was no match for the two louts who, having kicked and beaten him, pushed him down a grassy bank towards the canal. Rolling down the bank at an ever-increasing speed, Daniel was unable to prevent himself falling into the chill waters of the canal. Because of his childhood experience he had never learnt to swim and, being early evening, there was no one else in sight. Even the two youths who had attacked him had by now disappeared from view.

At this point I could see that Maxine was beginning to breathe more quickly and that she was becoming restless. I spoke to her, telling her to do as we had earlier discussed and detach herself from the scene so that she could see it and tell me about it but could not feel any distress, whether mental, physical or emotional. She sighed, then relaxed again and continued with her story.

Being unable to swim and with no one around to rescue him, Daniel had drowned in the canal that evening. However, it was not so much the fact that his life had ended which seemed to affect Maxine. Still detached from the actual sensations, she described how he had gone under the water and then come to the surface again several times before finally drowning. In fact, the water of the canal was not particularly deep and, had Daniel not panicked, he might even have been able to save himself.

I then took Maxine's mind off what had happened by asking her to describe again the scenery in the area of the canal and the painted barges and sturdy horses which had so fascinated the young boy. When I was quite certain that she was totally relaxed and comfortable, I brought her out of the regression and out of the hypnotic state.

The root of the phobia

As we discussed all that had occurred, it was quite easy for Maxine to see how her own phobia had been created. There was the experience for Daniel of falling in the water at a very early age, followed by the frequent admonitions of his anxious parents. Then there was not simply the death by drowning but the addition of the pain and violence which had preceded it. Most significant of all was the feeling of panic as the young man repeatedly sank beneath the surface of the water and then rose again during his last moments.

I asked Maxine what she felt about the session she had just experienced. She told me that once again she was convinced that her life as Daniel had been a real one. Because she had been detached from it at the most traumatic moments, she had not been caused any distress but was well able to see how the combination of Daniel's various experiences could have led to her phobia about water. She told me that she was relieved to know that there was a reason for it, even if the root cause had occurred so long ago. Maxine confessed that there had been times when she had thought she might be going mad, so great was her horror of water. Now she knew that, although the phobia had not yet disappeared – or even decreased – it had a basis in reality and not in some malfunction of her own mind.

The follow-up treatment

I had already explained to Maxine that discovering the reason for the phobia would not in itself be a cure, and that we would still have to work together to overcome it. She readily accepted this and was anxious to begin treatment right away. However, I suggested that it would be better for her to come back after another week as this would give her time to think over all that had happened, to listen to the cassette if she wished and to continue to practise her relaxation and visualization techniques. In any case, the phobia had been around for so long that one extra week would not really make any difference.

Maxine came to see me again the following week and we began the follow-up treatment, along the lines of those which you will find detailed in the 'case histories' sections of this book. It took four visits (over a seven-week period) to put an end to her phobia once and for all and to allow her to lead the happy, normal life she so desired.

4

Present-life Regression: The Original Experience

Now that you have a clear idea of what regression therapy involves, it is time to look at the sort of problems that cause people to need such therapy – why and how such problems have arisen in the first place and how they can limit people's lives and potential.

Parental influences

When a healthy baby is born, it does not come complete with sundry fears, phobias and personality problems. Those are only acquired as the baby grows up and travels through life. In many cases other people play a significant role in the acquisition of those problems – although not always deliberately. Sometimes the most doting and caring of parents can so overwhelm their child with protectiveness and a stifling form of love that they do not allow that child to develop. Perhaps they are so anxious for everything to go well for their offspring that they insist on making all his decisions for him. The result of this is that, when he becomes an adult, he is likely to experience a considerable amount of difficulty in standing on his own two feet – let alone taking responsibility for his part in the bringing up of a family of his own.

Sometimes, of course, deliberate cruelty is shown towards one or more of the children in a family – and such cruelty can be either mental or physical. We tend to think of cruelty as incorporating violence, but equally cruel is the father who constantly belittles his son or daughter in front of others. This naturally leaves considerable scarring on the personality of the child, just as beatings would do on his body. If this mental scarring is not treated in some way, whether by hypnosis or some other means, then the effects will last literally for the whole of his life. Indeed, those effects may well go on for generations, as a troubled parent will often produce troubled offspring of his own. For example, it is a recognized fact that a child who has been regularly beaten by one or both of his parents is extremely likely to inflict the same violence on his own children.

When dealing with cases of sexual abuse perpetrated upon a child, one of the greatest problems is the guilt which that child always feels during and after the event. Sometimes this is because the perpetrator himself has repeatedly warned his victim not to say anything, or he or she will either get into trouble or be disbelieved. The child, from his or her position of vulnerability, will accept this and will often keep silent – sometimes for years. Regression enables the former child to look back at the situation through the eyes of the adult he or she has now become and to see the reality of it all. From the adult position it will be clear that he or she was not in fact guilty of anything but that someone in a position of strength and power was taking advantage of his or her vulnerability mentally as well as physically.

Having observed his or her own former situation by means of regression, the patent will then during the course of a counselling session have the opportunity to discuss what happened (something that may never have been done before), to express anger at the perpetrator and possibly at others who may have guessed what was going on but perhaps did nothing to prevent it, and to understand that he or she was in no way to blame for what occurred. It is also helpful to know that he or she was by no means alone and that many others suffered in the same way. So, although it is tragic that every therapist is now hearing more and more from their patients about the way they were abused in the past, the fact that it is being brought out into the open and talked about publicly does bring some relief to those who until recently thought that their case was an isolated one.

Another reason to be grateful for all the publicity and discussion about child abuse is that former victims are seeking treatment at a far earlier age than was previously the case and therefore are able to go on and live a normal life once that treatment is complete. The patients whom I find most tragic are those who come for help in dealing with abuse which occurred fifty or sixty years ago, and which has often crippled them mentally and emotionally ever since.

The slings and arrows of life

In other cases it is a combination of circumstances or traumatic events which bring about the troubled state of mind. And quite often those events are completely beyond the control of the child himself, or even of the adults around him. It is easy to think of obvious examples: the child who suddenly loses both parents in a car accident; the outbreak of war, necessitating a dramatic change of surroundings and circumstances; a house fire or some other disaster befalling the family. Any of these is quite traumatic enough to cause long-lasting and damaging effects upon the mind of the child and yet each event simply 'happened' and there was no way that those caring for the child could have prevented it.

How we are influenced by others

Whether we think it or not, we are all affected greatly not only by our own hopes and desires but by hopes and ambitions that other people have for us. It is easy to think of the doctor, for example, whose father and grandfather were doctors before him and who takes it for granted that his son will follow in his footsteps – without really stopping to consider whether that is what his son wants to do. And if that child is sensitive and caring and does not wish to hurt or disappoint his parents, perhaps he may even enter the medical profession and spend years doing something he does not really want to do while denying himself the opportunity of fulfilling his life in the way he would have chosen.

The victim syndrome

Very young children think of their parents (or those who stand in that position) as 'wonderful' people who can do no wrong. Even the poor little mites who are physically or sexually abused do not, while still young, place the blame for such behaviour on the adult who perpetrates it. They will inevitably feel that it is their own fault – that they are in some way 'bad' or deserving of such treatment. When such children become adults they suffer considerable internal conflict. If they are able to remember the unpleasant incidents of their youth, their logical mind tells them that it was wrong and that the abuser was at fault. Their subconscious mind, however, has not progressed beyond the guilt stage and they continue to see themselves in their inner mind as bad people who deserve nothing better than to be victims. In many cases they are not able to remember anything at all about the earlier incidents and so all they have are those inner feelings with nothing to counteract them.

Because we all try to twist circumstances in such a way that they conform with our subconscious picture of ourselves, those who see themselves as permanent victims will automatically seek out people who are going to treat them as such. They will not know that they are doing so – but that is what will happen.

Rejection

It is not only the victims of mental or physical abuse who grow up with a faulty self-image. If the child feels rejected for any reason, that too has a traumatic effect –

whether the rejection was real or imagined. Because very young children have this inherent feeling that their parents can do no wrong, should one or other of those adults disappear from the scene for any reason, the child will always think that it is his fault.

It is not only the child of a broken marriage who feels this, but even when, sadly, one parent has died or spent a considerable amount of time in hospital. Indeed, many of those children whose fathers went off to fight in the war experienced that same sense of inner rejection, even though as they grew older they were able to understand the truth of the matter.

Put very simply, what the child feels in his sub-conscious mind is this: 'If this wonderful human being really loved me, he (or she) would want to be with me all the time. The fact that he has chosen to go away and leave me means that he does not love me. Because he cannot be wrong, that must mean that I am unlovable.' It makes no difference that the parent may not have wished to go (during the war) or may not have had a choice (death). The child's subconscious reaction remains the same and, unless careful understanding is given to him at each stage of his growing up, he will spend the rest of his life in such a way that he reinforces that self-image which tells him that he is not worthy of receiving love.

The conditioning of inheritance

There are so many ways in which we are conditioned by people or events that impinged on our early lives. Just as it is possible to inherit blue eyes or red hair, we can also inherit good and bad influences – both physical and mental.

Certain diseases are hereditary (or at least familial); sadly, it is being discovered that some babies are born already addicted to heroin or with the AIDS virus. Whether we inherit our temperament from one or other of our parents or whether we absorb it from prolonged contact is not certain. A recent research project has certainly proved that a large number of very young babies would stop crying or even go to sleep whenever they heard the introductory music to certain television soap operas. The theme tune of 'Neighbours' is particularly effective! This is not as ridiculous as it might at first seem. Most pregnant mothers are told to relax and put their feet up at some point every day – and many of them had done so while watching these television programmes. The baby inside the womb, therefore, had come to associate a particular signature tune with a peaceful and relaxed time, and had continued this association even after birth.

A child is also conditioned by anything he hears constantly. If little Jimmy's mother tells everyone that they can never go on a long journey because little Jimmy is *always* car-sick, then you can be sure that little Jimmy always *will* be car-sick. In the same way, a thoughtless parent who informs his or her child that he is 'stupid' will often be responsible for producing an adult who, even if he does not honestly believe in his heart of hearts that he is stupid, certainly does not have any real faith in his own ability. One of my former patients, whose ex-husband had spent their entire marriage telling her that she was 'stupid' or 'brainless', told me that, although she knew perfectly well that this was not true, by the time she had heard it said every day for the twelve years they had been together she had begun to believe that there must be something in it.

We cannot change what has gone; we cannot undo the wrongs others may – albeit unwittingly – have done to us. But, by regressing to the original occasion and examining the circumstances involved, we can gain sufficient insight into ourselves and our problems to prevent the past having a traumatic effect upon our present and our future. It is true that additional therapy may be necessary to achieve this end, but that therapy alone, without the preliminary understanding afforded by experiences during regression, would be an uphill task and might never work at all.

5

Present-life Regression:
Case Histories

Recall

Because we never actually forget anything but store it all
in our mental filing system, hypnotic regression can be
used to bring back both good memories and bad. In an
experiment conducted several years ago, students were
shown a short documentary film and, when the film was
over, they were asked twelve questions concerning what
they had seen. Most of the students were able to answer
most of the questions but, as you would expect, many of
the viewers had one or more questions to which they
could not remember the answer. Two weeks later the
same students were called together and reminded of the
questions they had been unable to answer. Then, under
hypnosis, they were regressed fourteen days to the time
of the showing of the film and they were able to watch it
again *in their minds only* – but this time, of course, they
were aware of the questions in advance and so they knew
what they had to look out for. At the end of the session
every one of them was able to answer the hitherto un-
answered questions. They had not been shown a repeat
of the film – they had merely watched it in their minds.

The incident with the students and the film was for
experimental purposes only. But such 'action replay' can
have a far more serious undertone.

Some time ago I received a frantic telephone call from
Carol, who had undergone successful hypnotic treatment about two years earlier. Her voice was shaking as

she told me that on returning from the cinema a couple of weeks earlier she had been grabbed from behind, dragged into an alley and viciously raped at knifepoint. The police had been called and, following her description, a young man had been apprehended.

The reason Carol contacted me was that she was now frightened to go out of her house, even during the daytime. She came to see me, and after two sessions, was able to overcome the problem.

I heard nothing more until a year later when Carol came to see me again. She told me that the trial of the young man was to take place the following month and that she was, of course, the only witness. The problem was that she had completely blocked the details of the incident from her mind. She knew what had happened but she had completely forgotten the details – including the description of the perpetrator. In some ways she was happy that she had no conscious memory of the details, but unless she was able to recall them she knew that there would be no case for the young man to answer and he would go free. And she was determined that this would not happen. She asked me whether I could help her to remember the events of that dreadful night.

I knew that it was quite possible to help Carol remember everything that had happened, but I also knew that it would be quite distressing for her – as indeed the trial itself would be. I also wondered how the police would feel about 'hypnotic memory-jogging'. As it turned out, the police officer concerned told us that, provided the details Carol remembered under hypnosis tallied precisely with the details she had given immediately after the crime, there would be no problem. As for Carol herself, she was quite prepared to recall the incident if it meant that it would help to convict the rapist.

I regressed Carol to the night of the crime, taking her back to the outing to the cinema rather than straight to the heart of the distressing incident. Because it is possible to turn the regressed patient into an observer rather than into someone undergoing the experience she was able to tell me everything that had happened in precise detail. She described the young man – what he was wearing, the colour of his eyes, the tattoo on his arm.

Once a regression is over, the patient is always able to remember all the details perfectly clearly, and for Carol it was more upsetting afterwards than during the regression itself. But she was pleased to have reawakened that memory, however painful it might be. In fact, she had probably done herself a great favour as, had she continued to suppress the memory, she might have caused herself great emotional problems in the future.

The details recalled by Carol during the regression (and which she continued to remember afterwards) tallied precisely with those she had given to the police on the night the rape had occurred. She was able to repeat them at the trial of the young man – and he was sentenced to seven years in prison.

Guilt

Myra was an elegant young woman of thirty-three with a successful career in advertising. To look at her you would have thought that she had her life perfectly in control – but how wrong you would have been. Myra sobbed as she told me that, although many men were attracted to her – and she to them – as soon as the relationship reached the stage of even the most innocent physical contact, such as a gentle kiss or even holding hands, something in her forced her to draw back and run away from the situation. She could not bear any form of contact with a man under any circumstances. And yet, much as she enjoyed her career and would not want to give it up permanently, she had a great desire for a strong, loving relationship and wanted to have children of her own – something she would never be able to do if her present feelings persisted.

Myra told me that, until the previous year, she would have thought that nothing whatsoever had occurred in her childhood which could have caused her revulsion to physical contact. Her parents had been warm and affectionate people and, as far as she could remember, she had been quite happy as a child. But about a year ago she had begun to remember incidents which she must hitherto have blocked from her mind.

When she was eight or nine years old, Myra had spent part of the summer holiday with her grandmother, who lived in a old schoolhouse in a small country village. Also staying there was her cousin Hugh, a boy of thirteen whose parents were travelling abroad. Hugh was a pupil at a boarding school in the north of England.

One day Hugh came into the bathroom while Myra was washing and offered to give her a present if she would give him a hug and a kiss. In her innocence Myra had complied with his wish and was rewarded with some sweets. This happened on several occasions, with the kisses and hugs becoming longer and more passionate as time went on. The little girl was not worried or frightened, being unaware that there was anything unusual in her relationship with her cousin. But things progressed from there, and Hugh began to ask her to take her clothes off and to let him touch her. Still Myra did as he asked. It was only when he asked her to come with him to the bushes at the bottom of the garden – something which she did willingly – and tried to force her to have sex with him that Myra became frightened and ran away. She never told anyone what had happened; soon afterwards the holiday came to an end and she returned to her family home. On the few occasions on which she and Hugh had met since that time, neither of them had ever said a word about that holiday.

Because, for the past twelve months, Myra had been able to remember these facts, she could not understand why her difficulties about relationships still persisted. She knew that Hugh had been wrong in what he had tried to do, but she also knew that no real intimacy had taken place. She wondered whether there was something else that she had blocked from her conscious memory

53

which was affecting her feelings towards men. She had read about the benefits of regression, and asked me whether she could go back to her childhood and try to uncover any other hidden details which might be relevant.

When Myra was regressed she was unable to come up with anything which might have had a distressing effect upon her before the incident with her cousin. So I took her through that holiday in greater detail. The only difference was that, until that final encounter when she fled from her cousin and his suggestions, she had been very willing to comply with all his wishes and, indeed, had thoroughly enjoyed the experience of being hugged, kissed and stroked by him.

Because, while being regressed, the patient is well aware of his or her present-day persona in addition to the previous one, Myra found it very distressing to think that she had been so happy to go along with all Hugh's demands. As an adult she was able to see how wrong it was and she knew that they were indulging in something they should not have been doing – although in her childish innocence she had not been aware that it was anything more than an extension of the love and affection she felt for other members of her family.

This had been the whole crux of Myra's long-term problem. It was not the intimate physical contact with her cousin which upset her, but the fact that subconsciously she felt so very guilty because she had enjoyed it so much. Although she was astute enough to understand this on a logical basis, it took several sessions of counselling and therapy to convince Myra's subconscious mind that she was in no way to blame and that she had behaved naturally and in total innocence.

Phobias

FEAR OF BIRDS

When treating a patient suffering from a phobia, I do not always regress them. In fact, I often leave it to the patient to decide whether it is necessary. As mentioned earlier, it is possible to treat certain phobias (although not all) by hypnosis without ever having to discover what caused them in the first place, and for some patients this is all they require. As long as the problem departs, they do not really care why it first arose. Others, however, feel very strongly that they *must* go back and discover the original cause – and, if that is how they feel, I will always go along with their wishes.

Joyce was just such a case. A middle-aged woman and mother of three teenage children, she came to consult me because she suffered from a phobia about birds. Over the past few years, that phobia had been getting worse. It was no longer just that she did not like birds or could not bear to touch them – she could have coped with that, as it would not have intruded greatly on her everyday life. But it had progressed to the stage where she could not make herself walk past a pigeon on the ground, but would cross the road in order to avoid it. From there things had grown even worse, and now she felt a sensation of panic if she even had to go to the local shops, in case she encountered a sparrow or two pecking at some crumbs in her path. Apart from the fact that she felt extremely foolish, her fears were now actually affecting her life and she felt that soon she would not be able to leave the house at all.

The regression itself took place on Joyce's second visit; the first was used to teach her deep relaxation. Having taken Joyce gently back through her childhood, we reached a time when she was just a toddler. She recalled an occasion when she was being taken for a walk in the park. She told me that she was wearing a blue hat and coat and that she was safely strapped in her pushchair.

Once in the park, Joyce's mother had stopped to talk to another young woman while Joyce herself sat watching some birds pecking at the remains of a sandwich that someone had dropped on the path. All at once one of the birds – it seemed enormous to the child, but may well have been as small as a sparrow – flew into the air and fluttered past the pushchair, its wings actually brushing the little girl's face. She in turn tried to get away from the bird, but was so firmly strapped into the chair that she was unable to move. Her mother had not noticed the incident and only turned to see what the matter was when Joyce began to scream. But, of course, by that time the bird – which was probably just as frightened as the child – had flown off.

That simple incident was enough to form the basis of the very real phobia from which Joyce was to suffer throughout the years which followed. It had not always been as bad as in the past year or two, but this is not uncommon as any form of fear or negativity feeds upon itself as time goes by. Perhaps as a child Joyce simply knew that she did not like birds and felt uneasy if one came near her. But soon she would have reached the stage where she would deliberately avoid going to places where birds were to be found at ground level – such as the local park. Each time she made a decision to keep away from birds, she was in fact reinforcing and enlarging the fear in her own mind, so that she changed from being someone who simply did not like birds to becoming a person who would actually consider spending the rest of her life within her own four walls rather than risk encountering a few sparrows in her path.

Now that Joyce knew and understood the reason for the onset of her phobia, it was not difficult for us to work together to help her overcome it. On her next visit to me I hypnotized Joyce, encouraging her to relax as much as possible. I then asked her to imagine that she was walking along a familiar street in her own neighbourhood. Ahead of her – quite a way in the distance – she could see some birds pecking at crumbs on the pavement. She then had to visualize walking slowly towards them, knowing that she could stop whenever she wanted to so that she did not feel that she was being compelled to go near these birds. At the same time I reminded her that she was feeling comfortable and relaxed and completely free from tension.

I asked her to tell me when she reached the point in the imagined scene where she felt she wished to stop walking along the street. To my surprise she felt able to walk right up to within a couple of feet of where the birds were. I asked her whether she felt she could walk past them, giving them as wide a berth as the width of the pavement would allow. She told me that she felt she could do this, and proceeded to do so. Although her breathing became a little faster as she imagined this part of the scene, she did not become noticeably distressed in any way; in fact she told me that she felt really pleased with herself for the way in which she had handled the situation.

The hypnosis session over, I suggested to Joyce that she should run through exactly the same set of images at least once every day for the next two weeks. She was to be sure to concentrate first on the relaxation part of the exercise, and was to stop immediately if she felt herself becoming at all upset.

When I saw her again two weeks later, Joyce couldn't wait to tell me what had happened. After she had been practising her exercise for about ten days, she had gone out intending to walk to the local post office. On her way she encountered two fat pigeons gobbling the remains of a dropped sandwich on the pavement in front of her. Not only had she managed to walk past these birds, but she had done so without experiencing the usual sense of panic. In the days since her visit to me, her mind had become so used to the idea of walking in the vicinity of birds that it had seemed quite a natural thing to do.

I asked Joyce what aspect of her phobia she felt still remained and she said that she would like to be able to go into an open space such as a park, where there were likely to be many more birds around.

Using exactly the same technique, I encouraged her to imagine doing just this and to practise for a further fortnight, after which she was in fact able to go to the local park and sit on a bench watching the children at play. She did not actually concentrate on the birds which happened to be there, nor did she feel any desire to feel them or encourage them to come near her – but she was quite able to relax knowing that they were there in the background.

Having completed her treatment, Joyce would never be a person who actively *liked* birds. But they no longer bothered her, and certainly they were no longer responsible for making her a potential prisoner in her own home.

CLAUSTROPHOBIA

Sylvia had been trying for years to overcome her claustrophobia, but with little or no success. Occasionally she was able to force herself to go in a lift if it was one of those with a window at the front so that she could see the passing floors. But more often than not she would climb the stairs – however many flights there might be – as she felt panic rising within her as soon as she tried to step into the lift.

Although she definitely did suffer from claustrophobia, Sylvia was by no means the worst case I have seen. She could not cope with lifts, and she could not go into the garden shed in case the door closed upon her. She would not travel on the underground or in an aeroplane, and felt panicky if she went into a department store and was too far from the door or windows. But I have had patients who were so badly affected that they could not travel in any enclosed vehicle – car, bus or train – had to leave the bathroom door open while they bathed, could not enter a cinema, theatre or even a small local shop. This affects not only the sufferer's life but also, of course, the lives of friends and family. Holidays become difficult, if not impossible. And in Sylvia's case there had certainly been causes for distress. She broke down when she told me that her little boy (now six years old) had asked every year to be taken to see Father Christmas in a nearby store, and every year she had had to disappoint him.

Sylvia was an intelligent woman, quite sensible enough to realize that there was probably some reason in her early life for the current problem. And yet, however hard she tried, she could think of nothing particularly

58

traumatic. True, she had been a baby at the time of the war, but her family had moved out to the countryside and their locality had never been troubled by bombing or anything else which might have caused her phobia. In fact she had been luckier than many. Because of a long-standing health condition, her father was not considered physically suitable for the armed forces and so he worked in a munitions factory not too far from their home. So, unlike many children at the time, Sylvia was fortunate enough to have both parents close at hand.

She told me that her parents had been kind and loving and that, when her two younger brothers were born after the war, she had got on with them quite well apart from the normal childish disagreements. Both her parents were dead now, but she was still in close contact with her brothers and their families and the relationship was a good one. Neither of her brothers was in any way afflicted by claustrophobia.

Using the techniques which I have already described I regressed Sylvia to early childhood – beginning, as always, with a remembered happy occasion. In this case she went back to her third birthday. Now the modern Sylvia realized that the family had very little money at that time and that the birthday party given for her was probably quite a meagre affair compared with the boisterous celebrations on her own children's birthdays. But little Sylvia had no thoughts of money; she was delighted with the cake and jelly and with the child-sized table and chair her father had made for her and the knitted doll from her mother.

One interesting fact emerged from her description of that birthday party, however, when she was describing the games that she and the other children played. Under hypnosis Sylvia remembered being adamant in her refusal to join in a game of hide and seek, which would have involved her in hiding in isolated, cramped and possibly dark surroundings so that she would not be found. Clearly her phobia was already in existence at that early stage in her life.

I decided at that point to begin using the detachment technique (see p.26). Going back slowly, a little at a time, it became evident that Sylvia's fear of being closed in had originated very early indeed; it was already established by the time she was one year old. We finally arrived at an event of which the adult Sylvia had no recollection whatsoever, but which to the baby must have been dramatically traumatic.

When she was about ten months old, baby Sylvia was lying in her cot in the house while her mother was busy in the kitchen. Her father was away at work. Now, although no bombs ever fell in the country district where they lived, from time to time the air raid warning sirens would sound and Sylvia's mother would take her baby and make her way to the shelter at the bottom of the garden, remaining there until she heard the 'all-clear'.

On this particular occasion, having picked up her baby daughter, the mother was in such a haste to reach the safety of the shelter that she tripped on the stone steps leading down into its dark interior. Falling down the steps, the poor woman banged her head against the side wall of the shelter and lost consciousness. Because she rolled over as she fell, the baby landed on top of her and so was cushioned from any physical harm. But the combined effect of the fall, the darkness and the feeling of being shut in and alone in this cold, murky world while her mother lay still and silent on the floor was sufficient to cause Sylvia acute distress. And it was that distress, outwardly forgotten, which had been the root cause of her lifelong claustrophobia.

When the regression was over, Sylvia expressed amazement at what had been revealed. She had never known anything about that occasion; her mother had never mentioned it – and had certainly not seemed to suffer any ill-effects herself. Sylvia found it strange that her mother had never connected the incident with her daughter's later distress at being in closed-in places, but I pointed out to her that the awareness of the link between early incidents and later emotional problems was a comparatively recent phenomenon. Having experienced the regression, she could easily understand that such a distressing early occurrence could be the cause of the phobia which followed.

It is interesting to note that, although Sylvia was able to recall the events of that fateful afternoon and to describe in great detail the sights, sounds and emotions which prevailed, she had no idea at all of how long the two of them lay on the ground before her mother regained consciousness. She could not tell whether it had been a matter of minutes or several hours. This, however, is not at all uncommon when regressing someone to such an early age, for babies do not have an awareness of time in the same way that adults do.

Although this regression had given Sylvia insight into the initial cause of her claustrophobia, it was not sufficient in itself to put an end to the problem. We still had to go on, in the way I shall describe later in this chapter, to deal with that aspect of treatment. Yet a great deal had actually been achieved. Having established that there was a genuine reason for her phobia, Sylvia no longer felt stupid or guilty about it. In addition I explained to her that, having found the original event and looked at it through adult eyes, there was no danger that she would put an end to one problem only to replace it with another, as might have happened if we had not investigated its origins.

Even when the basic cause of a present-day problem comes to light early in the regression session, I never go on to the follow-up treatment during the same consultation. It is better by far for the patient to have a week or so in which to mull over all that has occurred and everything he or she has learnt about the past. In the course of that week the facts become simply a matter of personal history and the enormity of the problem later caused is somehow minimized and put into proportion. The prospect of a cure no longer seems impossible to believe, however long the patient has lived with the problem itself.

Follow-up treatment: first consultation

Sylvia rushed into my room on the occasion of her first follow-up session, so anxious was she to get started on her treatment. Of course this demonstrates another advantage of regression therapy; by the time the patient starts the treatment itself, he or she has already become used to how it feels to be hypnotized and has confidence in the technique as well as in the therapist concerned.

We spent a short time discussing how Sylvia now felt about that long-ago event and whether it caused her any distress to think about it. There was absolutely no problem here. Because it had taken place so long ago and was one of those things which could happen to anyone, she was quite unconcerned about the accident itself. In addition, having had several days in which to think about it, she could see quite clearly how it had been responsible for the problems which had been harassing her all her life.

So, having no more to discuss on that topic, I went on to ask Sylvia if she could think of a place in her own home where she felt uneasy if the door was shut. There was no hesitation in her reply. Like many homes, her house had a cupboard under the stairs where things like suitcases and cleaning items were stored. Sylvia was able to take from the cupboard only those items she could reach while standing in the hall itself. Anything deeper in its dark interior had to remain there until another member of the family could get it out for her. The fact that her husband had fitted an electric light inside the cupboard made no difference at all; it was the thought of being within that cramped space – even with the door to the hall left open – that Sylvia could not bear.

I then asked her whether she would be prepared – in the safety of my consulting room and under my guidance – to imagine standing inside the cupboard and closing the door. I reminded her that, since she would be doing this under hypnosis, it was still possible to use the detachment technique if I thought she was becoming distressed in any way. Thanks to her acquired confidence in what could be achieved in the hypnotic state, Sylvia readily agreed.

Having guided my patient into a state of hypnotic relaxation, I asked her to imagine that she was indeed standing in the hall of her own house, just outside the cupboard under the stairs. Then I asked her to visualize taking hold of the doorknob and pulling open the cupboard door. None of this caused any problem at all as it was something Sylvia was well able to do in reality.

Then she had to imagine switching on the light in that cupboard under the stairs and taking a couple of steps forward so that she was just inside – but with the door open to the hall and with the knowledge that she only had to take a single large step back to be out there again. As I made these suggestions to her, I was continually reminding her that she was feeling very relaxed and comfortable and that she was in complete control of the situation and need do nothing (even in her imagination) that she did not choose to.

When she had visualized standing just inside the cupboard, I asked her how she felt about it; she replied that, so far, she was feeling quite at ease. I then suggested that she take small steps, one at a time, further into the depths of the cupboard – remembering that this was all in her imagination and that she was still feeling totally relaxed. She was to tell me what she was doing and to stop as soon as she wanted to. Slowly she imagined taking one step after another until she reported that she could physically go no further because the slope of the ceiling was so steep.

Now I asked her whether she felt able to imagine switching off the light in the cupboard, still leaving the door open to the hallway. I reminded her that, if she felt it necessary, she could use the detachment technique and simply observe herself doing as I suggested. However, she said that she was quite happy to visualize the scene without having to detach herself from the reality of it.

After about thirty seconds, I told her that she could switch the light on once more and make her way out of the cupboard and back to the hall. I then brought the session to an end by bringing her out of the hypnotic state.

When I asked her how easy or difficult she had found the exercise, Sylvia told me that she had been quite surprised at how simple it had been. In the past she had only to think of being in an enclosed space and she would feel panic rising within her. But the peaceful feeling which accompanies hypnosis and the constant reminders that she was relaxed and comfortable and everything was simply happening in her imagination had served to prevent any fear and anxiety at all.

Now came the opportunity for Sylvia to play a significant role in her own treatment – something which I consider vital if the cure is to be permanent. She was going to have to do some regular 'homework' in order to reinforce the suggestion in her own subconscious mind. Every night – in that twilight time which comes between being awake and falling asleep – Sylvia was to lie in bed and spend some minutes concentrating on relaxing her mind and her body and establishing a regular breathing pattern. Then, knowing that she was safely tucked up in her own bed, she would go through the mental exercise as she had done under hypnosis and imagine herself entering that cupboard under the stairs. If at any moment she began to feel tense or anxious, she was to stop and concentrate on making her body relax once more before returning to her visualization.

Then I suggested that, *when she felt ready to do so*, she should try to carry out the exercise in reality rather than simply in her imagination. But she was not to force the pace in any way. There was no 'correct' length of time which should elapse before she was ready to try, so it did not matter how long it took. Once she had managed to enter that cupboard successfully without any fear or panic, she was to telephone me for another appointment.

Twelve days later I received a call from an exultant Sylvia who told me that, on the previous evening, she had in fact managed to go right into the cupboard and switch off the light. She had even pulled the door to – although she had not closed it tightly. And, what is more, she had not experienced a single moment of panic during the whole exercise. She could hardly believe it, and she could not wait for her next consultation to see what was going to happen next.

What had happened to change Sylvia so drastically during the course of twelve days? Why did she not experience the usual terror at being shut in a small enclosed space? And can it really be so simple? All these questions came tumbling out the moment she entered my room a couple of days later.

What Sylvia had accomplished while doing her home-work was to convince her subconscious mind that she was quite capable of entering an enclosed space without fear; and since it is the subconscious which is responsible for sending out all those panic signals – the racing heart, the sweating palms, the feelings of nausea and so on – those symptoms did not appear. You see, your subconscious mind cannot tell the difference between what is real and what is imagined; so, although the information it had received during those twelve days was in fact a product of Sylvia's imagination, the effect on her subconscious was precisely the same as if it had been actual experience. For twelve days her subconscious mind had 'seen' Sylvia calmly and confidently entering the cupboard under the stairs with no signs of panic; so when, on the thirteenth day, she came to do it in reality there was still no need for anxiety to manifest itself. And after she had succeeded in doing it once, Sylvia began to reverse the whole process so that those signs of panic would never appear again.

Another way of looking at it is to think of an actor who rehearses and rehearses his lines in order that his perfor-mance may be as near perfect as possible on opening night. Sylvia had been repeatedly rehearsing her chosen situation for twelve days so that, when she made the actual attempt on the thirteenth, her performance too might be perfect. But, even while visualizing entering the cupboard, she had at the same time been fully aware that she was in a non-threatening situation (lying in her own bed) and so, once again, the subconscious mind had no need to send out those panic signals.

Just as failure often follows failure, success breeds success. Sylvia's problem had arisen in the first place because of the negative situation imprinted on her subconscious memory when her mother lay unconscious in the darkness of the air raid shelter. But now, rather like recording afresh over the existing programme on an audio or visual cassette, Sylvia had superimposed a successful situation and had thereby made a significant change in the data recognized by her subconscious.

Follow-up treatment: second consultation

Once I had discussed the situation with Sylvia and explained to her what had been happening, we were able to progress to the next stage. Having dealt successfully with the dreaded cupboard under the stairs, we had to find another situation for Sylvia to cope with. This time I left it up to my patient to decide which area of her life was causing her the most distress. Although she was anxious to be able to travel on the underground and in aeroplanes, she felt that the problem which caused her the most inconvenience was her inability to go into any large shop or department store without experiencing extreme panic. She did not find it too difficult to go into a small shop – say, the local newsagent or the greengrocer at the corner of the street – as she was never too far from the window or the door. But it was years since she had felt at ease in any store which went back a long way from the street and therefore had no windows through which she could see daylight.

This seemed a suitable area on which to work, and we proceeded in precisely the same way as before, with Sylvia imagining the situation under hypnosis and then going off to do her homework for however long was necessary. This time she contacted me again after just a week to say that, for the first time, she had been able to buy clothes for her children in a certain famous store rather than having to rely on ordering from a mail order firm.

Follow-up treatment: third consultation

This was the last time I needed to see Sylvia. She was now so convinced that the technique worked that she was quite able to deal with other situations on her own, using precisely the same methods. On this occasion I hypnotized her, stressing heavily not only the relaxation but also that she was now in control of her life and could use what she had learnt to overcome feelings of claustrophobia in any given situation.

Some months later I received an emotional telephone call from my happy former patient. She was calling me from central London, having travelled there with her young son on the underground train. It was the first time she had been able to grant his wish and take him to visit Santa Claus in a large department store, and that made it for her the happiest Christmas she could remember.

This same technique can be used for patients suffering from any type of phobia. It does not necessarily work as quickly as it did in Sylvia's case – but it *always* succeeds, provided the patient does his or her homework regularly and conscientiously. The number of days of practice needed before the patient has the courage to try and translate the visualization into action varies considerably, not only from one individual to another but even as regards the different stages of a person's treatment. I have known patients who took three or four weeks to accomplish the first stage but who managed the second within a day or two. Others have progressed rapidly in the beginning, only to experience considerable difficulty in overcoming the final hurdle – almost as though the mind was loath to give up a fear to which it had been clinging for years. But I have rarely known a patient need more than four sessions of hypnosis after the discovery of the original source of the problem.

Stammering

Clive had a stammer and had learnt through regression that it had originated when he had been the subject of bullying at school. However, that knowledge was not sufficient to rid him of the problem, so we continued the treatment by using hypnotherapy.

Follow-up treatment: first consultation

Using my normal methods, I hypnotized Clive; he was such a tense young man that I was grateful that he had already experienced regression. Because a regression session is longer than one involving simple hypnotherapy, the patient tends to relax more and more as the session goes on. This made Clive much better able to relax during the course of the follow-up treatment. A bonus was that he had been so fascinated by his earlier experience that his confidence in hypnotherapy as a whole had grown, and he was far more willing to undergo treatment than he might otherwise have been.

It is an extraordinary fact that anyone who stammers because of an earlier traumatic experience loses the affliction when hypnotized. So one of the first things I did with Clive after hypnotizing him was to ask him simple questions – 'What is your full name?', 'Where do you live?', and so on. He was able to reply to each of these without stammering once. I then asked him to sing a line or two from a song (it could be anything from a nursery rhyme to a pop song), which he was also able to do successfully. I recorded all this on audio cassette; when the session was over, I played the tape to the astonished Clive who had been so relaxed when hypnotized that he had not even realized that his stammer had temporarily disappeared. Although this knowledge was by no means sufficient to put an end to the stammer, it did help to convince him that the problem was capable of being solved.

I then spent some time trying to teach Clive how to breathe! It is surprising how many people go through life breathing inadequately and, although in many instances this does not prove to be too great a problem, in the case of someone with a stammer it can increase their difficulties enormously. Everyone, when tense or anxious, breathes both too quickly and less deeply. The person whose stammer is caused through lack of confidence or chronic anxiety is breathing this way for the greater part of the time. When you exacerbate this situation by confronting him with direct questioning or something which intimidates him and causes him to feel even more nervous, his breathing can become so rapid and so shallow that it borders on hyperventilation. Therefore, even if he did not have a stammer, there would not be enough breath in his lungs for him to speak his words properly.

So the remainder of the first consultation was spent showing Clive how to breathe from his diaphragm rather than from the upper part of his chest. His homework for the coming week was to practise his breathing exercises twice a day and to listen to the cassette of himself speaking under hypnosis without the trace of a stammer.

Follow-up treatment: second consultation
Clive practised his exercises diligently and, when I saw him the following week, he had mastered the breathing technique – although it still took a great deal of concentration on his part and was not something he did naturally. In addition, having listened repeatedly to the cassette he felt much happier in himself, realizing that the stammer which so embarrassed and distressed him was not going to prove incurable.

Once Clive was in the hypnotic state on this occasion, I asked him to visualize going up to someone he knew slightly, taking a few deep breaths and then asking them a simple question – 'Could you please tell me the time?' or 'Do you know the way to such-and-such a street?' Within this visualization everything would naturally go well. He would be calm and unafraid and, because he had remembered to breathe deeply before starting, he would ask the question in an easy manner without stammering at all.

It was important that, to begin with, Clive was to approach only people whom he already knew by sight – even if he had never actually spoken to them before. There was no point in asking him to practise on his parents or his sister as, although still in evidence, his stammer was far less noticeable with members of his own family. Equally, no purpose would have been served by asking him to approach total strangers in the street, as the mere thought of this would have been so terrifying to the young man that he would probably have given up there and then.

Just as Sylvia had eventually to translate her visualization into reality, so too did Clive. I suggested that he wait until he felt ready, and then try actually asking a simple question of someone he felt would be approachable, and finally to telephone me once he had achieved it.

Clive had an extra piece of homework, too. Once a day he was to practise his relaxation technique and his breathing exercise and then, in the privacy of his own bedroom, to try reading aloud from any book he chose. If (as I expected would be the case) he was able to accomplish this with very little in the way of stammering, it would go even further towards increasing his self-confidence.

Follow-up treatment: third consultation
It was about two weeks later that I saw Clive again. He came into the room with a broad grin on his face and could hardly wait to tell me that not only had he managed to approach several people at work and ask them questions, but that he had decided to put himself to the test over the last few days and had, in fact, gone up to complete strangers in the street to ask them the time. In addition, his reading aloud had proved to be successful except for a couple of occasions when he had had a particularly stressful day and had found it exceedingly difficult to relax. However, he was able to see the reason for the added tension on those days and not to allow that to interfere with his overall progress.

Feeling of failure

In general we are our own worst enemies when it comes to enlarging and reinforcing our fears, so that what may have begun as a minor apprehension can escalate into a problem of mammoth proportions. And the initial events do not have to have occurred way back in our childhood – last year will do. Perhaps it is the fault of the world in which we live, but people seem to have a great fear of failing, forgetting that failing at something does not mean that one is a 'failure' at life. Indeed, it is from our failures that we learn our most valuable lessons. And every human being has the right to fail; it is what he or she makes of that failure which counts. How many people do you know who failed their first driving test? They did not all give up there and then, but presumably went on to take the test again and eventually to pass – many of them at the second attempt. And there are many men and women who, having 'failed' at a first marriage, have gone on to learn from that failure and to have extremely happy second marriages. If each of those people had said, 'I am a failure. I am no good at marriage', they would have deprived themselves, their subsequent partners and possibly their children and other relatives of much happiness in the future.

Over the years many men have come to my clinic because they have considered themselves failures in one vital respect. They have become impotent – a fact which naturally causes a great deal of anxiety to them and to their wives. Before I can take on such a patient I naturally ask him to consult his doctor to ensure that there is no physical cause for the problem. Once this has been confirmed, we can assume that the sudden loss of sexual ability has a psychological cause.

This is a problem which seems to affect a considerable number of men in their forties and fifties, at a time when there may be a good deal of pressure on them at work and at home. While some of them are able to accept the situation with equanimity and wait for it to pass, others tend to panic and assume that the condition must of necessity be a permanent one. Of course, matters are not helped by the fact that many men have difficulty in talking about the problem at all, often finding it both distressing and embarrassing. And, indeed, this distress may be sufficient in itself to prolong the situation.

71

Looking at it logically, it is not particularly unusual for any man, particularly if he is tired or has had a little too much to drink, to be temporarily unable to achieve an erection on a single occasion. Provided he does not allow himself to panic, the matter usually ends there. For those who do become anxious, the problem arises the next time he wants to make love. Instead of the moment being one of passion and desire, his mind is often filled with such thoughts as 'I hope it doesn't happen again' and 'Please let it be all right this time'. Those thoughts in themselves are sufficient to turn the occasion from a loving one into some sort of physical test – and of course the same thing happens again; the man feels so tense and anxious that he is simply not able to perform sexually.

Now of course he has two failures to build upon. And this is what he frequently does. Logic does not come into it at all. Suddenly a man will see himself as a sexual failure rather than as someone who simply had not been able to achieve an erection on one single occasion. And, however much his wife or girlfriend tries to reassure him, eventually he begins to feel that his very manhood is in question.

Any intelligent man, once he has been given the opportunity to voice his feelings, will understand just what he has done and be able to see that it makes no sense at all to build upon an isolated failure when he has a lifetime of 'successes' about which he could think. By means of regression it is possible to take such a man back to one of those occasions when his own and his partner's mutual desires had culminated in a very happy and successful sexual encounter for them both.

The next part of the treatment is to ask him to visualize such a situation over a period of a week or two while, at the same time, trying to refrain from the sexual act itself – although kissing and caressing his partner, whether in bed or not, is to be encouraged. What usually happens is that, because the pressure to succeed has been removed, before that two weeks has elapsed the couple will find themselves overcome by the passion of the moment and a joyous and successful sexual encounter is likely to result.

Anyone who suffers from a phobia or from any of the other problems mentioned above encounters all sorts of difficulties in their everyday life. For one thing, they often feel that they must hide their condition in order not to appear foolish in the eyes of others. For, whereas everyone can see the sense of avoiding deep or rough seas, fewer people can understand the unhappy individual who is so terrified of water in any form that he or she cannot even bear to wash their hands.

Personal confidence is not something which stands still. Just as positivity breeds positivity, negativity breeds negativity. The individual who is calm and self-assured is far more likely to perform well in his chosen area of life, even though he may not necessarily be the one with the highest level of ability. You have only to think of such ordeals as driving tests or interviews. The majority of candidates who fail do so because they have been so nervous that they have not been able to think clearly, far less to perform well. And, if you think about it, all that the would-be driver has done is to use his mind and his imagination to visualize all those things which could possibly go wrong and cause him to fail.

If negative visualization can be so effective, there is no reason why the positive and creative use of the imagination should not be just as effective. But, of course, it rarely works like that. It is bad enough to fail one's driving test once; to do so for a second time reinforces the sense of hopelessness in the learner's mind – he now has twice as many failures to build upon – so that he uses his ability to visualize in an even more negative fashion. And so it progresses. From being someone who simply happened to fail his first driving test, he becomes a person who '*always* goes to pieces when sitting beside the examiner'.

Bearing all that in mind, it is not difficult to see how the person who starts with a lack of confidence in one specific area of life soon seems to be taken over by that lack of confidence, which spreads to many spheres of activity. The longer the problem goes on – and many of my patients have suffered for years – the worse it is likely to get. And every time a patient tries unsuccessfully to *force* himself to overcome it, his sense of failure merely adds to the general feelings of inferiority and so his confidence drops even further. To make matters worse, because he always does fail in his attempts to improve the situation, the sufferer convinces himself that he has nothing to look forward to but a lifetime of misery.

There is one other significant point to be remembered, and that is that the person who suffers from what appears to be an illogical fear *always* feels that he or she is stupid. In fact, this is probably one of the commonest ways in which patients describe themselves. They are often fully aware that their problem has no basis in present reality and so, because they are unable to do anything to overcome it, they believe that they must be stupid. And the longer the situation continues and the greater the number of vain attempts at dealing with it, the more stupid they feel. Being able to look back, by means of regression, and discover that their condition has a logical and rational cause, takes away that feeling of stupidity and prevents the patient condemning himself to a lifetime of inevitable failure.

Building on small successes

There are very few people who have never achieved any form of success in their lives. This does not have to have been the winning of some special prize or coming first in every race. It is quite sufficient to find something of which the individual concerned is proud – however small and seemingly insignificant that something may appear to be.

One woman told me that it was the day she was able to swim the width of the local pool after years of being afraid. For another it was learning French at evening classes when she had always been considered a complete duffer at languages. Success is such a personal thing. If you have grown a beautiful rose, learnt to type or finished the *Times* crossword, you have succeeded in something which mattered to you.

When working with the patient who considers himself a consistent failure in a particular area of his life, part of that treatment may well involve regressing him to the time of one of these earlier successes. In this way he can re-experience the *feeling* of succeeding and may accept that he is capable of that feeling and of having achieved something by his own efforts. When this acceptance is combined with positive visualization, the cycle is often broken so that past fruitless attempts play no further part in the prospect of future achievement.

Some years ago I worked with a golfer who had achieved a considerable amount of success, winning several amateur trophies. Peter first came to see me halfway through the golfing season. He could not explain it, but his putting had gone to pieces for the past few months and he was missing shots which formerly he would have holed with ease.

I do not play golf, nor do I have any particular interest in the sport, so there was nothing I could teach Peter in the practical sense. But there were two things I could do. First, I regressed him to former years and previous golfing tournaments when he had done exceedingly well, so that he was again able to savour the feeling of success and achievement. Next we worked together on using his imagination to help him visualize putting the ball from any position on the green and watching it roll gently into the hole.

Because Peter was already an experienced golfer he knew just how he should stand, how he should hold the club, what sort of swing was required and how hard to hit the ball. He had lost none of his ability – it cannot suddenly disappear without physical cause. All he had lost was his confidence – his belief in himself. Once we had worked together to help him regain his faith, he was able to go on to play just as well as he had done before; indeed, now that he had remembered the feeling of success, he was able to play even better.

Dealing with presumed 'stupidity'

'I know I'm being stupid!' These were Kirsty's opening words to me the first time I saw her. And yet she was certainly far from unintelligent. An attractive young woman in her mid-twenties, she had been just one year away from her final examinations as a solicitor when, two years earlier, she had been rushed into hospital for an emergency appendectomy. The operation had apparently been quite straightforward; Kirsty was home in under a week and back at work after a month, with no obvious after-effects. Since that time, however, she had never been well.

No one could identify the problem – indeed, the symptoms varied considerably and seemed to travel from one part of her body to another. She had been prodded, probed, examined and X-rayed on numerous occasions, but no cause for her ill-heath could be unearthed. Eventually she had been sent to a psychiatrist to see if he could help discover the reason for what appeared to be a purely psychosomatic condition. But this too came to a dead end. No one could find out why this apparently healthy young woman suffered symptoms which were so intense and yet so varied.

Then one day Kirsty met an old friend who happened to have consulted me in the past for regression therapy. This friend suggested that there might be something which had happened at an earlier stage in Kirsty's life which was causing her health to deteriorate now. Feeling desperate and willing to try anything, Kirsty finally came to see me one day in early spring.

Calmly and concisely she related her history to me. Her logical mind told her that there was absolutely nothing wrong with her physically, and yet scarcely a day passed when she did not feel unwell or suffer some unidentified pain. It was for this reason that she called herself 'stupid'.

Since all had been well before Kirsty went into hospital to have her appendix removed – and since many people have a very real terror of hospitals in general – I decided to regress her to that particular time. Under hypnosis she was taken back to the first day of her stay in hospital – the day before the operation itself. Although she told me she was experiencing a certain amount of discomfort due to the condition of her appendix, and although she was not really looking forward to surgery and to the anaesthetic, none the less Kirsty seemed to have no more than the expected apprehension which would have been felt by anyone.

I then took her forward slightly to the evening after the operation, a time when she was fully awake and over the more drastic effects of the anaesthetic. I asked her how she felt now. To my surprise Kirsty burst into tears. No, she told me, she was not in any great pain – simply the discomfort she would have expected to follow surgery. She was not aware of feeling particularly ill. It was just that she *knew* that there was something seriously wrong with her – something far more dramatic than a grumbling appendix or the normal after-effects of an operation. Oh, the doctors and nurses had assured her again and again that she was fine and would soon be fit and well again. And yet, as she kept repeating, she was convinced that there was something that no one was telling her.

Since Kirsty had been feeling quite confident before the operation and yet that feeling had disappeared immediately after surgery, it seemed that something must have taken place in the theatre itself. Now I had never before tried to regress anyone to a time when they were under the influence of anaesthetic, but I decided to do so on this occasion. And the effects were more dramatic than I could have imagined.

Kirsty was able to tell me a great deal of what had taken place in the operating theatre. She could not feel anything at all – the anaesthetic having done its job – and she could not see anything as her eyes were tightly closed. But she could hear! She described the sound of footsteps, the noise of theatre machinery and even the sound of the instruments being handed to the surgeon. But, most significant of all, she was able to hear and understand every word which was spoken.

Conversation consisted mostly of routine theatre talk – the request for instruments or comment upon the operation itself. At one point she was aware of two nurses speaking about an outing they were planning with their boyfriends. But then it happened. She was aware of a new sense of urgency in the theatre and she heard a female voice saying: 'I think we're going to lose her.' This was followed by the voice of another woman: 'Even if she survives, she'll never be right.' And there was silence apart from the sounds of the operation itself and the clipped tones of the surgeon as he gave his orders. Finally it was all over and Kirsty heard the instruction being given to take her to the recovery room.

All this was information that Kirsty revealed to me during the course of the regression session while she was under hypnosis. Until then she had had absolutely no recollection of anything which had taken place in the operating theatre. She had certainly never thought that her long-term health – or even her life – was under threat. All she had been told when she came round after the anaesthetic was that there had been a few complications and the operation had taken rather longer than had been expected.

Whatever the complications may have been, and whatever those theatre nurses may have thought, the fact was that Kirsty had suffered no physical ill-effects once she was over the post-operative period. But now, at last, she was able to understand why all those psychosomatic symptoms had arisen plus the general feeling of being unwell. Her subconscious had registered and clung on to those unfortunate comments made during the course of the operation. Deep in her inner mind, therefore, Kirsty believed that something terrible was going to happen and that her health would fail.

Once the amazing facts had been revealed to Kirsty during the course of her regression, she only needed to come and see me one more time. On that occasion we began by discussing mistakes and human fallibility. We agreed that the man or woman does not exist who had never made a mistake, however foolish. There is no champion tennis player who has never served a double fault; no professional musician who had never played a wrong note; and no doctor or nurse who has not made an error of diagnosis.

After this discussion I hypnotized Kirsty and took her back once again to the time of her operation. This time, of course, she was not only armed with the fore-knowledge of what would be said but she still had in her mind the conversation we had just had about making mistakes. Once again she was aware of the sounds in the operating theatre. Once again she heard the nurses discussing their social life and then those thoughtless comments which had been responsible for instilling such negative thoughts in her subconscious mind. Only this time she was able to tell herself that 'Anyone can make a mistake' and that these two nurses were, in fact, wrong in their hasty prognosis.

During the course of this session, I repeatedly reminded her of the fact that she was seeing something which had happened some time ago and that time had proved her recovery to be complete – something which had been born out by the numerous examinations and X-rays she had since undergone.

Inheriting fears from others

When we are young we are greatly affected by those around us – not simply by what they do but by their attitudes and beliefs. It is patently obvious how a fear which is openly expressed can be passed on. You have only to think of the situation in which a mother is terrified of thunder and panics whenever she hears it, rushing to close the curtains and to cower in the corner of the room. Naturally that is bound to affect a child, particularly if that child is sensitive by nature. To see a parent – someone he thinks of as being all-powerful and ever-capable – reacting in such a way must induce in the child the belief that whatever it is that is causing such terror must be dreadful indeed and that he, therefore, should be equally terrified. Thus are the seeds of future panic sown.

Sometimes the adult can try so hard to hide a fear that the very effort seems to emphasize the apprehension. When I was very young, I was bitten on my face by a dog. For many years afterwards I was naturally very wary of any dog and, although I soon learnt not to run away, as this would only make them run after me, I never willingly approached them. By the time I had children of my own, I had overcome by fear to a great extent but I was still a little nervous. I was determined that I would not communicate this nervousness to my sons, and so I did my best not to react should we come across a dog in the street. And yet both my sons, neither of whom had ever been hurt by a dog, would show apprehension if a dog approached. Indeed one of them would insist on crossing the road rather than walk past the animal. So in some way I must have passed on my fear to my children, even though I thought I was doing everything in my power to avoid doing so. (I an happy to report, however, that none of us now has any fear at all of dogs – indeed familiarity has made us quite fond of them.)

Because all human beings are fallible, with individual fears and weaknesses, it is so easy for the foundation for a similar fear in our children to be laid even when we think we are doing our best for them. Think how much worse things can be when a thoughtless (or, even worse, a malicious) adult comes into contact with a vulnerable child.

Traumas caused by words

If the way adults act towards a child can have a traumatic effect on their lives, so too can the way they speak. It is impossible for any of us to monitor carefully every single thing we say – how boring and stilted our speech would be if we did – but it is as well to remember that young children take the spoken word very literally, and a great deal of harm can be caused by the use of thoughtless and insensitive phrases. We are all aware of the damage that can be done by threatening to 'call a policeman' or 'fetch the bogeyman', but many more casual phrases – never intended as a threat – can do just as much harm.

One former patient told me how her early childhood had been marred by her mother forever threatening to 'walk out and leave you all to it' whenever there was any family dispute – or even when one of the children did not comply with a request quickly enough. It was only as the girl grew older and she realized that her mother was simply mouthing words and had no intention whatsoever of carrying out her threat that she had begun to be able to relax and enjoy what was left of her childhood. However it had had the effect of making her very careful, after her own children were born, about the way she spoke to them.

Eileen suffered a similarly induced trauma. She was sent to me by her doctor, whom she had consulted because she suffered from anxiety attacks and what she called 'turns'. These involved being unable to breathe properly, and on occasions even caused her to faint. They did not seem to follow any particular pattern, but occurred at random and with varying intensity. She had had every test her doctor could think of, had been seen by a senior consultant and even by a psychiatrist, but no one could find a reason for the attacks. In the end the doctor, being far-sighted enough to believe in the value of hypnosis when properly practised, sent her to me to see if between us we could unearth the cause of the problem. (I would point out at this stage that I would

81

never begin to treat a patient with physical symptoms of this sort unless he or she had first consulted their doctor and was able to tell me that no physical cause for the problem could be found.)

Apart from the distressing nature of the problem itself, Eileen was most upset because she felt it was ruining her whole life. She was an Irish Catholic woman of twenty-eight and had been married for nearly two years. She wanted desperately to start a family – and not just to silence the constant enquiries of well-meaning friends and relatives. But she was afraid to allow herself to become pregnant and therefore, although it was against her religious beliefs, was using contraceptives. This in itself caused her to feel guilty and so added to the distress she already suffered.

She had two main reasons for fearing pregnancy. The first was that she was afraid that she might have an attack while pregnant and would cause some harm either to herself or to the unborn child. The second reason was that, even were she to have a successful pregnancy and birth, she was terrified that she might one day be carrying her child in her arms when she fainted and might then drop or hurt the child in some way.

To begin with, I tried the relaxation and controlled breathing techniques which usually prove effective in counteracting panic attacks – but to no avail. The greatest impediment we encountered was the lack of a 'trigger' in Eileen's case. It is often possible to identify situations which immediately precede anxiety attacks of this sort, and so the patient is forewarned and can take preventive action. In this particular case, however, there was no such conformity; the attacks seemed to occur at random intervals and in many differing situations.

Unable to think of anything else to do, I suggested to Eileen that we tried regressing her to her childhood. She agreed, but pointed out that she had had a very happy childhood, being the youngest of eight children in Ireland. There had never been a great deal of money, but no one had ever gone hungry and the feelings of warmth and love between the members of the family had more than made up for the lack of luxuries.

When I regressed her, Eileen did in fact describe to me a happy, boisterous childhood with her sister and her six brothers – all of whom took great delight in spoiling their baby sister. Eventually we came to an occasion when Eileen was about four years old, the only one of the children not yet at school. It was a warm, sunny day and she was playing in the garden while her mother was hanging out the washing. She recalled asking her mother – in the way that youngest children often do – whether they could 'buy' another baby for her to play with. Her mother answered her, using a phrase that so many people unthinkingly use, by saying that they were not going to have another baby because 'After all, it nearly killed me having you.' This was not in fact true. Eileen's mother was a strong healthy woman and had not suffered any particular ill-effects at the birth of her youngest daughter. One can well understand, of course, her lack of desire for another child when they already had eight to feed and clothe, and naturally she can have had no idea of the effect on Eileen of her casually spoken words. But they did have a drastic effect. They instilled in the subconscious mind of the little girl an absolute terror of pregnancy and childbirth, linking them irrevocably with thoughts of death.

When not in a regressed state Eileen had absolutely no recollection of those words being spoken by her mother. Indeed, she could not even remember the day in question or her request for a baby to play with.

What Eileen had done, of course, when she reached the stage in her life when she might naturally have been considering starting a family, was subconsciously to 'invent' her illness in order that she might be spared the horrors of it all. She had not done this deliberately; she was not even aware that she had done it. She had not been able to imagine why she should be suffering those anxiety attacks for so long. But, although she had progressed from happy childhood to happy marriage, all the while a conflict was raging within her. On the one hand, as a good Irish Catholic girl married to a man she loved and who could afford to support her, she felt it her duty as well as her wish to have a child. On the other hand, the little girl locked within her subconscious mind still linked thoughts of childbirth with her mother's comment that it 'nearly killed me'. Had she merely stated that she did not wish to have a baby, she would have been considered failing in what she saw as her role in life. The panic attacks gave her the perfect excuse, as no blame could possibly be attributed to her. The adult Eileen was quite intelligent enough to understand the devastating effects of those careless words on the child she had been – although she did not blame her mother in any way for using them.

Because the panic attacks had become a habit with her, I spent a few sessions with Eileen teaching her how to overcome them. It was not very long before she was free of them altogether. I do not know whether she went on to have a family – but I do know that there was now nothing to prevent her doing so.

6

Past-life Regression

Mention the word 'reincarnation' to any group of people and you will probably be astounded at the number of different reactions you will get. On the one hand, there will be those whose belief in the concept is so definite and so fixed that they almost allow it to rule their lives. In the opposing camp you will find the dyed-in-the-wool sceptics who cannot even begin to conceive that perhaps there is something in it. And, lying somewhere between these two extremes, you will find almost every shade of belief – or perhaps of hope.

Most people inhabit this in-between land, perhaps not fully accepting the concept of reincarnation but none the less thinking that 'there must be something there'. Perhaps they have had an experience of déjà vu which they cannot explain by any other means. Perhaps they have read or heard of some of the research which has been done in this field in recent years, and it has opened up their minds. Perhaps they just find it comforting to think that this one earthly life is not the beginning and end of it all.

Personal reincarnation, of course, is something which it is impossible to prove or disprove, although theories and beliefs abound. But if you think that such a belief is necessary in order for a patient to gain benefit from past-life regression therapy, you are wrong – as I hope to be able to explain in this chapter.

There may be many reasons why a patient under hypnosis is able to experience past-life regression (or, as the doubters might call it, 'flights of fancy'), but any of them can play a significant part in the overcoming of that patient's particular problem. There are three main theories, described below.

Actual regression to a previous life

Just for a moment, suppose that it had been proved beyond doubt that reincarnation was a fact and we all lived not just once but many times. And suppose that in a previous existence you had suffered a particularly unfortunate fate – let us say that you met your death in a burning building. Would that fact not help to explain the presence of a phobia about fire in this lifetime? Remember that a phobia is an illogical fear and not simply the natural caution with which we all treat potentially dangerous substances such as fire. And it is this very illogicality which causes the phobia sufferer to feel foolish or inferior – particularly if the unnatural fear is of something which others would consider harmless. If the phobic now has an explanation for his or her terror and an actual experience on which to base it, the feelings of stupidity disappear. Of course, it is still necessary to proceed with therapy to help overcome the fear itself, but no barrier of inferiority or failure has to be overcome.

Ancestral memory

Jung expressed the view that, although recall does in fact exist, what is happening when regression to a previous life appears to be taking place is that the subject is simply tapping into some vast communal memory bank, and it is from this source that he obtains his information. I understand this theory and, while I am not able to disprove it, I feel that, in the light of all the research which has been done in more recent times, it leaves too many gaps which no one has yet been able to fill.

Imagination

The sceptics will tell you that, because there is no such thing as reincarnation and therefore no such thing as regression to a previous life, the whole thing is a figment of the subject's imagination.

Let us accept this third theory for a moment and agree that, when a patient under hypnosis experiences what appears to be a past-life regression, he is in fact making the whole thing up. If this is true, ask yourself why he should do so? It cannot be simply for the fun of inventing fairy tales about himself. By the time a patient comes to consult me (or any other professional therapist for that matter), he is aware that he has some sort of problem in his life and that he wants to get to the bottom of it. He also knows that, since therapists have to eat and support their families just like everyone else, it is going to cost him money to do so. It would be a foolish and expensive form of self-indulgence to pay for a course of treatment just for the pleasure of making up fancy tales about previous incarnations. So we can probably rule out the theory that he is indulging in a weekly exercise in make-believe.

This leaves us with the possibility that, while the previous life the patient describes may not actually have happened, he is not deliberately inventing it but relating something which may have been created in his subconscious mind and which he really believes to be true. I accept that this is a possibility and that, even if one believes in reincarnation, there may be times when it is the patient's subconscious which is providing the 'information' about a previous existence. But does this make it play a less significant role in overcoming his problem?

Take the example of the person with an illogical fear of fire. Does it matter whether he really died in a burning building or whether he only thinks he did? The effect is the same. Reliving the experience (even if only in his imagination) will still take away his feelings of foolishness and will provide him with a reason for his phobia. From that point onwards, treatment will be the same.

The subconscious mind is not haphazard in the way it works to protect you. If it creates a set of images in your mind (whether real or imaginary), there has to be a reason for the selection of that particular set of images as opposed to any other.

When Barry came to see me, he was suffering from physical manifestations of what was obviously a great deal of pent-up aggression. We could find no cause for this when I regressed him to an earlier period in this life and so I went on to regress him to what appeared to be a previous life. Then things were very different. He described to me a life of violence and hatred in which he lost no opportunity to vent his anger upon those around him – and, what is more, he actually enjoyed doing so. When the regression was over, Barry was able to see that, because of his past experience, he had become terrified of showing even the slightest sign of aggression in this lifetime in case he once again lost control and reverted to his former self. This understanding went on to form the basis for his ensuing therapy, involving both visualization and counselling, which proved highly successful and relieved poor Barry of the symptoms from which he had been suffering.

I hope this helps you to see that it does not matter at all whether that regression to his past life was factual or whether Barry's subconscious had caused him to invent the whole thing in his imagination. The happy outcome would have been precisely the same in either case.

My own beliefs

I think at this point it would be a good idea to tell you what my own personal beliefs are – and please remember that I am not attempting to convert anyone else to them. The very essence of the word 'belief' is that it is a conclusion based upon thought and experience but one which cannot be irrefutably proved.[1]

I believe that reincarnation exists and that it is possible for an individual to tap into a previous existence by means of regression. When I first began the work that I am doing now, I decided to keep an open mind about the topic; but, as time has progressed, I have been able to record details of fact, time and place given to me by my patients which have later been checked and confirmed and found to be wholly accurate. These are not the kind of facts which can be found in the history books; they are small matters which would be of no real importance except to the people concerned.

One of my former patients – an antique dealer from Chesterfield in Derbyshire – was regressed as part of his therapeutic treatment. During the course of that regression he told me his name, his trade (he was a cloth merchant) and the fact that he lived and worked in the Bristol area. Some months later, after his treatment had ended, he wrote and told me that, during his summer holiday, his curiosity had led him to visit Bristol and its surroundings – and he had had the somewhat strange experience of finding his former name on a Parish Register in the district of Yate. Now the name was not a famous one, the cloth merchant having lived his life in the comparative obscurity common to most of us, and my patient had never before visited that part of the country – and yet the details he unearthed coincided perfectly with the facts he had given me during his regression.

DÉJÀ VU

Many people have had experiences of déjà vu, when they have come across a place which they are able to describe

---

1. When I talk about 'I' and 'my' experience, I do not intend in any way to detract from the findings concerning previous lives revealed in their researches by people far more eminent than I am. But, although you will find some recommended reading in the bibliography, I decided to relate only what I have encountered during the course of my own work.

in precise detail even though they know they have never been there before. I know that such experiences are often said to be the result of the individuals concerned having read a book or article or seen a film or television programme about the particular place and then having forgotten that they have done so. But there are times when this theory just does not hold water.

A former patient (one who had never been regressed or even thought about the subject) told me of a strange incident in her own family. She lived with her husband and little girl in the city of Worcester. One day they were invited to visit some old friends who had moved to Hereford.

The family did not own a car and so they made their journey by coach. When they arrived in Hereford, they bought a street map of the area in order to find the road where their friends were living. The man remarked to his wife that they had to make their way towards a particular church and that, once they had found that particular building, they would be almost on their friends' doorstep. They consulted their street map but, before they could work out their route, the little girl told them that they had to go down the hill, over the bridge, past another church, turn to the right and they would come to the church for which they were looking. Her parents gazed at her in astonishment. How could their daughter know all this? She had never been to Hereford before, had never even met the people they were going to visit and – being just four years old and as yet unable to read – could never have learnt about the district from a book. And yet, when they followed the little girl's instructions, they did indeed find themselves outside the church which was to be their landmark.

It is often the case that children seem able to recall past lives (if that is what they are) more easily than adults. A great deal of fascinating research in this area has been done by Dr Ian Stevenson, one of the most eminent and respected workers in this field. Dr Stevenson, who at one time held the chair of neurology and psychiatry at the

University of Virginia Medical School, worked with children in India and other eastern countries; his findings are published in his book, *Twenty Cases Suggestive of Reincarnation*. The fact that the younger the subject is, the more able he is to recall details of past lives, seems to me to be quite simple to understand: it is only as our children pass through the Western educational system that they are taught to forego intuition and creativity in favour of logic and calculation.

THE PURPOSE BEHIND IT ALL

So, if I believe that we each have a number of incarnations, what do I think is the purpose of it all? Here again, because positive proof is not available, I can only offer you my own theories for your consideration.

I believe that each of us has what I term a spirit (but which I am quite happy for others to call the soul, the higher self, the inner self – or any of dozens of different names) and that it is this spirit which has a journey to make through several lifetimes. This is not just for the pleasure of travelling but for the purpose of learning and evolving. And in order to achieve this end, the spirit has to dwell within a number of different entities.

Think of life on earth as junior school and the spirit as the pupil. Just as each child has to learn a series of lessons and skills as he passes from class to class until he is ready to enter the senior school, so I believe that the spirit too is given a series of lessons to learn before it is free of earthly life altogether and able to progress in whatever is the equivalent of its senior school. Because I do not accept absolute predestination, however, and cannot believe that we human beings are simply pawns in some giant chess game being played in the wide blue yonder, I think that it is the person within whom the spirit chooses to dwell who actually makes the right or wrong decisions.

Let me give you an example. Suppose the lesson a spirit has chosen to learn in one lifetime is to renounce any form of violence. It is the human being who will be faced with the opportunity and perhaps the temptation to be violent, and who will make the decision as to which path to follow. If that decision is the right one, then the spirit can progress to the next lesson; if the person gives in to temptation, then the spirit has to be faced with that choice again and again (either later in that same life or perhaps in a future one) until the right decision is reached.

I accept that this is quite a basic and simplistic way of expressing what has to be a deep and complex theory, but the story of Martin may provide more clues.

SELF-AWARENESS

Martin was a local businessman who wanted to discover more about himself and, who as part of his treatment, underwent regression therapy. Over a period of about a year he was regressed six times at regular intervals. Although when regressed one does not go back to the immediate past life, then the one before it, then the one before that and so on, by the time Martin had experienced regression six times it was possible to put the lives in chronological order so that we could try and see if there was any lesson to be learnt from them.

When people such as Martin, consult me not in order to seek help in overcoming a particular problem, but to help them to understand themselves, their motivation and their spiritual journey better, I do not see the patient at weekly or fortnightly intervals but leave gaps of anything up to six or eight weeks between visits. During this time the patient has time to think about the latest piece of the 'jigsaw puzzle' and, in many cases, to meditate upon it.

It follows that people who are seeking this sort of help will undergo several sessions of regression. I suggest to them at the beginning of each session that they will learn about a different existence from any they may already have experienced. The greatest number of past lives experienced by any of my patients during the course of such discovery is eight – but this does not mean that we do not have far more than that, simply that the patient chose to stop after that number.

It was interesting to note that in each of his previous six lives, which ranged from the fifteenth century to the late 1890s, Martin had been given the opportunity to be a 'teacher'. I do not mean by that someone who stands in front of a class of children, but a person who is able to pass on wisdom and knowledge to others. These opportunities included being a member of a sixteenth-century religious order, an elder statesman and a doctor. In each of the six lifetimes concerned, Martin had in fact deliberately rejected that path and turned to something more materially oriented. And yet the same opportunity always re-presented itself, time after time.

Earlier in this twentieth-century lifetime Martin had trained to become a psychotherapist and counsellor. But he had given it all up and returned to the business world as a marketing executive.

I am not attempting to judge Martin in any way at all. He has every right, as we all do, to choose his own way of life. But, from a study of the pattern of his previous lives, it would seem that at some point – whether as Martin or at some time in the future – he will have to accept the role of teacher, guide or helper.

As you have read the above paragraphs, many of you will already be forming your own opinions – and this is just as it should be. All I ask of you in this, as in any other area, is that you keep an open mind. If I were to rewrite this book in ten years' time, in the light of further research and experience, my own views might well have changed somewhat. But all I can do at this moment in time is tell you where I stand today.

HYPNOTIC RECALL

People often ask why, if we are able to recall details of previous lives under hypnosis, we do not remember them consciously. But how confusing this would be and what a turmoil would exist within our minds. If previous lives do, in fact, exist, then everything we ever do or learn is stored in our subconscious. When our body dies, however, our conscious mind dies with it; so that, when the spirit enters a new body, it enters a new conscious mind with a clean memory-slate. The subconscious mind, as we have already seen, is protective in the extreme. We each absorb millions of pieces of new information as we progress through life; think of the confusion if this information became jumbled up with facts learnt in any number of former lives – and many of these facts would now, of course, be out of date because of the technological progress made by man.

Sometimes we are given glimpses of former existences – whether we recognize them as such or not. The person brought up in the city who has a natural and instinctive knowledge of the curative properties of herbs and wild flowers; the person who experiences déjà vu or the one who seems to recognize a 'stranger' although the two have never met before; the person born with talents he has not had time to acquire – is it not a possible explanation of the genius of such prodigies as Mozart that he actually brought with him skills and talents he had learnt in a previous lifetime?

MY OWN REGRESSION

When I was a child and had never even heard the word 'regression', I was always fascinated by anything to do with the Tudor period of English history. I would read every book I could find about it and became reasonably well-informed about the subject.

Some twenty-five years later, when I became interested in hypnosis and then in regression therapy, I began to wonder whether my earlier fascination was because I had actually lived in Tudor times. Later, when I came to be regressed myself, I was curious as to whether I would 'remember' anything of a Tudor existence. However I was also intelligent enough to realize that, because of my extensive reading on the topic, I was capable of inventing a pretty good story about life in that period. Had I been asked to imagine myself as I would have looked during that time, you can be sure that I would have had the beautiful gown, the ruffled frill and the bejewelled fingers of a lady. When, as part of my training, I was regressed under hypnosis by my late husband (also a qualified hypnotherapist), I did indeed turn out to have lived during the Tudor period – but I was a pig-farmer's daughter who, having lived a pitiful existence, died from a gangrenous leg at the age of fifteen. A comparative 'nothing' of a life, you might think; and yet it did more to convince me that it was not my imagination at work than all the finery of a court lady could have done.

Past-life regression by non-hypnotic methods

Of course, hypnosis is not the only method of inducing past-life regression. There are, in fact several others but, for various reasons which I shall attempt to explain, I do not feel that they are always quite as effective – or indeed as safe – as the use of the hypnotic state.

SPONTANEOUS REGRESSION

Although many people tell of brief experiences of déjà vu, spontaneous regression in any depth is somewhat rare. Even the validity of many of the 'I've been here before' experiences is rather doubtful as, with the growth of television and cinema, we have all seen so many places which we may later come to visit. But we may well have seen them without registering that fact; perhaps a film is set in a particular location and we are so involved in the plot that the background scenery enters only our subconscious mind. Then, when we actually visit that place for the first time, a subconscious memory is triggered and we are convinced that we knew instinctively what it would look like.

This does not mean that I do not believe in the existence of genuine déjà vu experiences – indeed I have already shown that I do. It is just that I believe they are probably more rare than is claimed.

The only people who are likely to experience extended periods of spontaneous regression are those who have been practising deep meditation over a prolonged period of time and have reached a high degree of competence in this field. Because deep meditation can be likened in many ways to the altered state of hypnosis, and because those who have a profound interest in such forms of meditation are likely to be on a deliberate spiritual voyage of discovery, they may be able to pass more easily through those barriers of protection normally erected by the subconscious mind. I do not feel that any harm will come to those people who experience spontaneous regression in such a way, as any group involved in the higher levels of meditation should be under the control of a qualified and experienced teacher or leader who will be on hand to control the situation and to help should the pupil find himself in emotional difficulty.

It is also possible to have what seem like experiences of past-life regression while dreaming. I have to say here that I honestly do not know whether such experiences are examples of genuine recall or figments of the dreamer's imagination. So many of our dreams, however, are mixtures of fact and fantasy that I do not feel any great reliance can be placed on what seem to be insights into our former lives when we are asleep.

THE CHRISTOS TECHNIQUE

This is a method of inducing a past-life regression which has the reputation of being safe and effective. It involves a combination of massage, meditation and visualization and is done with the aid of a helper. This helper first massages the feet of the subject, then the head, and finally guides him or her through a mental exercise intended to lead to the regression itself.

The background of this method is somewhat uncertain. It is thought to have originated in the United States and to have gone from there to Australia. The acknowledged current expert, G. M. Glaskin, has written extensively about the subject.

I have no personal experience of the Christos technique, but apparently it has achieved some interesting results including the ability of the patient to give a detailed account of a previous life. It does have certain points in its favour which are found in the hypnotic technique too, and which I consider vital in the interests of safety and authenticity:

- another person is present at all times, not merely to assist the subject to enter the regressed state but to help him avoid any difficulty or distress;

- the 'evidence' comes from the subject himself and is not given to him by another person.

PSYCHIC OR ASTROLOGICAL EVIDENCE

There are those who claim to be able to tell you psychically just who you were and what sort of life you had in a previous existence. There are others who claim that they can draw up astrological charts which will provide similar details. I am in no way decrying such methods – perhaps they work and perhaps they do not – but I do feel that they are open to considerable abuse. While I am sure that there may indeed be any number of genuine psychics and astrologers who can do precisely what they claim in this field, what is to prevent charlatans telling you that you were a Roman gladiator, a druid or even Napoleon? They cannot prove that they are right and you cannot prove that they are wrong. How much better it is when any facts or pieces of information come from you yourself. And, if we are looking at regression as a form of therapy – as, indeed we should be – the benefit can surely only come when you re-experience the previous existence for yourself (or even when you imagine that you do).

(I must tell here the story of a charming American lady who approached me when I had just given a talk on regression therapy. This lady informed me that she and her friend had consulted a man who claimed at that time to be the leading expert in the United States in the psychic determination of past lives. The two ladies had each paid 500 dollars for the privilege of a ten-minute consultation, during which one was told that she had been a quartz crystal in a former life while the other was informed that she had been an E flat! I make no comment.)

THE VALUE OF HYPNOSIS OVER OTHER METHODS

For many reasons I feel that hypnosis is by far the best method of inducing past-life regression:

1. There will be another person with you constantly during the session – one in whom you have confidence and who will be able to guide you gently into the appropriate altered state of mind.

2. Because there are various physical signs of impending distress when the subject is hypnotized, the therapist will be able to help you avoid any such emotion by using the detachment technique. In this way you will be able to relate what is going on while not actually experiencing it.

3. Any evidence, whether actual or a product of your subconscious, comes from you yourself and is not simply given to you by another person who might or might not know what he is talking about.

4. As well as the hoped-for benefits from the regression itself as part of a prolonged therapy, any hypnosis session involves deep relaxation and therefore the patient is able to release a great deal of accumulated stress and tension.

5. It is possible to go on with the same therapist to deal with the problems which caused you to need the regression experience in the first place.

7

Past-life Regression: Case Histories

Here are some case histories, taken from my own notes and records, which I hope will illustrate the therapeutic value of past-life regression – whether actual or an invention of the subconscious mind of the patient. All the facts are true; the only thing changed, as elsewhere in this book, is the names of the people concerned.

Failure to communicate

Some years ago a fifteen-year-old boy was brought to see me by his father. Paul was an intelligent and affectionate lad but he had suffered all his life from a severe communication problem. It was not like autism, where the condition is usually permanent; sometimes Paul was fine, but whenever he was asked direct questions he was physically unable to speak. The muscles in his throat would constrict and he could not utter anything more than strangled animal-like sounds. As if this were not problem enough, years of being shouted at and punished by teachers totally lacking in understanding had only made matters worse.

Paul's father told me that they had been to see specialists, speech therapists and psychiatrists in several countries and no one had been able to discover a reason for the boy's affliction. The only thing all these consultants had been able to agree upon was that the problem was purely psychological.

Paul was more than willing to undergo hypnotic treatment, as no one was more anxious for a cure than he. It was interesting to see that he had no difficulty whatsoever in answering questions while in the hypnotic state. This, however, is not unusual, as I have mentioned earlier. People with speech impediments which are psychologically rather than physiologically caused are able to enunciate clearly and well when in the altered state of hypnosis.

Once we had established the fact that Paul was able to communicate with me when hypnotized, I asked him if he would be willing to try regression therapy. Once I had explained the concept to him, he was anxious to proceed.

The first two sessions did not reveal anything of dramatic impact. This is not unusual, as the subject's subconscious is getting used to 'playing a new game' and, being ever-protective, will often not allow anything traumatic to occur. By the third session, however, Paul was becoming more at ease with the idea of regression and more confident about the technique itself.

During session three, Paul regressed to what he told me was a life during the Second World War. He claimed that he was an American pilot and that he had been shot down and captured in Nazi Germany. At that point all he would do was repeat to me, over and over again, a name, rank and serial number. Then he told me that he had, in fact, died during the course of the interrogation which followed his capture.

Now I know nothing whatsoever about the United States military, but I wrote down the details of the name, rank and serial number and gave them to Paul's father. He in turn checked the details with the American authorities and was told that there had been a thirty-two-year-old pilot who had disappeared during the war – the only record claiming that he was 'Missing, presumed dead'. But he had had the identical name, rank and serial number.

If there is no such thing as regression to a previous life, how was Paul (a fifteen-year-old boy from West London with no American connections whatsoever) able to give precise details of a pilot who was not famous in any way and who was probably known to no one but his friends and family? And, if that pilot died suddenly under interrogation, is it not possible that the reincarnated spirit would have brought with it a terror of questioning – a terror which manifested itself in a physical form? If the case of Kirsty (p.76) offered a dramatic example of what can be brought forward by the subconscious mind during the course of regression to an earlier time in present life, Paul's revelations must surely have been some of the most dramatic among patients who claim to have been regressed to a former existence.

It would be wonderful to be able to report that this revelation about his past was sufficient to bring all Paul's problems to an end and that he was then able to communicate fully and well with all those around him. Wonderful – but untrue.

But there was one very important benefit which Paul gained from that session. Once it was over, he told me of his great sense of relief when he realized that there was a reason for his condition and that he was not – as he confessed he had feared for most of his life – 'going mad'. Even had later sessions of hypnotherapy not helped him as much as they did, that fact alone would have been sufficient to have made his life far happier and, therefore, the whole exercise worthwhile.

Follow-up treatment: first consultation
The first thing we worked on was the physical constriction of his throat which Paul experienced when confronted by direct questioning of any sort. In the beginning, this type of condition is treated in a very similar way to Clive's stammer (see p.67). But because both Clive and Paul could respond well to me under hypnosis did not mean to say that they could react in the same way to others. However it did give them hope, because it showed them that they were capable of 'normal' speech, even though a considerable amount of work might be required to achieve this end.

I recorded a personal cassette for Paul which was not unlike those which form part of foreign-language courses. On it I asked him simple questions, ranging from 'What is your name?' to 'What is the weather like today?' (using some to which the answers would always remain the same and others to which they would vary). In each case the question would be followed by a pause long enough for Paul to give the answer. He took this cassette home with him and I suggested that he should use it at least once a day. First he had to relax in the way he had been taught and then, while still lying on his bed, he would listen to the questions and then answer them aloud. I explained that it might take several weeks before he was able to do this – after all, we were trying to undo the damage of fifteen years – but I was pleasantly surprised when he telephoned me after a fortnight to say that he could now do as I requested.

Follow-up treatment: second consultation
We now had to begin to work on a far greater problem, and that was Paul's total lack of confidence. Not only had he been tormented by his condition for the whole of his life, but he had experienced years of mockery at school plus the trauma of being taken from one doctor to another for as long as he could remember. These facts, understandably, had simply made matters worse by robbing the boy of any vestige of confidence he might have had. We had to work together to try and give him back the positive self-image to which he was entitled but which he had lost so many years ago.

A great deal of this second consultation was spent talking – a process which took far longer than one would suppose, because of Paul's difficulty in expressing what he felt. After all, this facility which most of us take for granted was something he had never had before. Just as I do with others whose confidence is at a low ebb, I suggested that initially we should select a comparatively small hurdle to overcome – although of course it would not seem particularly small to Paul himself. I asked him whether he could think of something he would like to be able to do but which, until now, he had felt was beyond him. I found his answer sadly touching. He wanted to be able to go into a café or coffee shop and order a drink for himself. Most of us take the ability to perform such an action for granted. But not Paul. It was not that he was incapable of asking for a cup of coffee or a soft drink; he was terrified that his request might be countered with a question ('Would you like milk or cream?', 'Do you want anything to eat?') and you will remember that it was questions which were the initial cause of his problem. So, rather than find himself forced into a position where he would have to deal with the embarrassment of unsuccessfully struggling for an answer, he simply avoided such situations altogether.

Once again that wonderful piece of equipment – the imagination – was to be the main tool in helping Paul to deal with the problem. Having relaxed him (something which was still not easy) and hypnotized him, I asked him to imagine the situation he had for so long avoided and to visualize going into a local café, sitting at a table and ordering a coffee. As part of his visualization, the waitress serving him was to ask whether he wanted a cup or a pot of coffee as well as enquiring if he would like something to eat. He was to see himself answering both questions simply and successfully – in fact, if he wished, he could actually speak his answers aloud while visualizing. Only when he was completely happy with this process was he to attempt to translate thought into action.

The outcome
This time only ten days elapsed before I heard from Paul again. It is not unusual when dealing with a child or adolescent to find that they progress in tremendous leaps, as opposed to the more cautious steps of some older people. Perhaps it is because a young person is more willing to accept the whole concept of hypnotherapy and regression, whereas older – and probably more sceptical – patients find it harder to accept something which they do not fully understand. Perhaps it simply means that the younger the patient the more

adept he is likely to be at using his imagination – he has not yet become so enmeshed in the logical and the mundane that he has forgotten how to see pictures in his mind. Of course there are exceptions to this rule, but younger patients do tend to respond extremely well to hypnosis in all its forms. And Paul was no exception.

Over the next few months Paul progressed extremely well, finding himself able to deal with situations which had formerly caused him both physical and emotional difficulty. Then we reached a sticking point.

During the time I was treating him, Paul had his sixteenth birthday and immediately begged his father to allow him to leave school. He had been so unhappy there and, in spite of his undoubted intelligence, his affliction had caused him to fail one examination after another so there seemed little point in forcing him to stay on. In addition, both teachers and fellow pupils had come to regard him as 'different' or 'odd' and they were either too busy or too insensitive to realize that he was, in fact, in the process of changing. So they continued to treat him in the same way as before, which did not do Paul's rather fragile confidence any good at all. So, all things considered, his father felt that he might indeed be happier elsewhere.

But where was he to go and what was he to do? Further education establishments seemed to be out of the question because of Paul's inadequate academic record and also because his unhappy experiences in school had made the whole idea of college a terrifying one. For a time he drifted from one mundane and unsatisfying job to another – filling shelves in a local supermarket, helping with the fruit-picking at a nearby farm and delivering handbills from door to door. While none of these jobs was either fulfilling or well-paid, at least Paul was able to prove to himself that he could do *something* – even though each time he was deliberately putting himself in a position where he had little contact with other people and would not have to deal either with questioning or with figures of authority.

Then, one day when he was delivering handbills, he found himself walking up the path of the local animal sanctuary. The superintendent, a caring but eminently practical woman, noticed the boy's curiosity and asked if he would like to come and see the animals. For Paul it was love at first sight. Now he knew what he wanted to do, and that was to help care for these unwanted and often neglected creatures to the best of his ability. Two days later he began working at the sanctuary. Because of his lack of knowledge and experience he was given the most basic tasks to perform, but this did not worry him at all. He was able to pour out to these defenceless creatures all the love and tenderness which had been bottled up within him for so many years and for which, until now, he had never been able to find an outlet. He still had very little money and no particular prospects – but he was happy.

Naturally I was delighted that Paul had at last managed to find his niche in life. It did mean, however, that his progress in one sense had come to a halt. He was generally much more confident in the everyday areas of his life and certainly within the job at the sanctuary itself. He felt more and more at ease with both the superintendent and the other staff who worked there – after all, they had a common purpose and a common sense of devotion to their charges. But of course he was now in a position where he did not have to answer questions – or even to talk much at all, so his actual progress in that direction had of necessity come to a halt, perhaps for ever. I discussed the matter with his father and with Paul himself and we decided that, certainly for the present, the plus factors far outweighed the minuses and that Paul's happiness and his ability to live a normal life were all that mattered.

The problem of unchanging attitudes

Paul's case also serves to highlight another difficulty faced by many patients when they are trying to deal with the problems in their lives. People around them have grown used to them and their ways and, however much the patients may try to change themselves, those people still tend to see them in their former light. If you are someone who has always gone to pieces when faced with any form of responsibility, and others have become accustomed to taking that responsibility out of your hands, then that situation is likely to continue even when you are working to improve yourself, and you may find it difficult to persuade them to give you the chance to show what you have achieved.

Paul's situation at school was made impossible because of the way in which he was seen by the teachers and by the other pupils. The changes he had struggled to make in himself were in doing things that these other people found normal and easy to do, so they were not inclined to give him any credit for his progress. In the end the only answer was for him to leave.

It is always difficult, when a patient is trying to build up his or her confidence, to know how to deal with this situation. It would probably be best if he could tell the more sympathetic among his family or friends just what he is trying to achieve and to ask them to let him know when he is making progress. But, of course, if you are someone with a very low self-image, you will not want to draw attention to yourself in this way.

In the beginning, therefore, many people have to be content with the knowledge that they are improving and – even more important – that they are doing it by their own efforts. It sometimes helps to keep a list or even a chart of your successes so that you can see in black and white just what you have achieved and can refer to it on those days – which will naturally occur – when you wonder whether all the effort is worthwhile.

Self-starvation

Alison's mother brought her daughter to see me because she thought that the girl was suffering from anorexia nervosa. Like Paul, Alison had done the rounds of hospitals, specialists, consultants and psychiatrists, and the opinion of all the experts was that this was not anorexia in the true sense.

Although anorexia is sometimes called 'the slimmer's disease', its roots go far deeper than a desire to lose weight. It is, in fact, a deeply rooted psychological problem which, as a general rule, only manifests itself in adolescent girls. (Boys, men and older women, whatever is generally thought, do not suffer from anorexia except on rare occasions – although of course there may be other psychological reasons, often linked to how they feel about their own sexuality, why they might choose to starve themselves to the point of emaciation.)

The true anorexic has a psychological fear of growing up and becoming adult; in many cases there is also an inner conflict between the girl concerned and her mother. This is not to say that the mother may not love her daughter and that everything she does may not be in what she considers to be the girl's best interests – but that conflict is there, somewhere beneath the surface. What the anorexic is trying to do by means of her starvation is to maintain the body of a young child – slight and slim, with no breasts and no periods – so that she does not have to face the world of womanhood.

I agreed with the other consultants whom Alison had seen that she did not fit into this category. But the fact remained that this young woman (who was just twenty-one) had a horror of putting on weight and an intense dislike of most foods. When I first saw her she weighed under six stone even though she was five foot seven inches tall.

In cases such as this, I always like to liaise with the patient's own doctor so that we are aware of what the other is doing. Alison was having regular check-ups and vitamin injections, as well as other treatment, and I insisted that she continue with all of this during the time we worked together. But, in the meantime, we would see if we could discover some underlying cause for her obsession.

Alison proved to be an excellent subject for hypnosis, being both intelligent and co-operative. (This, in fact, was another reason for deciding that she was not suffering from anorexia, as such patients do not really want to be cured and therefore respond far less well to hypnosis.) Having tried regressing her to earlier periods of her present life, we had been unable to come up with any trauma which might possibly account for her condition. She was quite willing to be regressed further so that we could see whether perhaps the cause was more deeply buried in her past (or her imagination, whichever you think it to be).

Looking for clues in past lives
Under regression Alison told me that she was a man called Jacob who had lived in the early part of the nineteenth century. She was able to give me clear and detailed descriptions of the town in which she lived, the clothes and way of life of the people, and her impressions of the surrounding countryside.

Now Jacob, as described by Alison, was an evil character who spent much of his life engaged in criminal pursuits – many of them involving violence. As he grew older, he seemed to enjoy inflicting pain upon others for the sake of it rather than simply for financial gain, as had formerly been the case. During the course of his miserable career Jacob was responsible for the deaths of several people – some by poisoning and others by strangulation. He was an altogether obnoxious character and it was fascinating to watch Alison as she relived the experience. One part of her appeared to delight in her own (that is, Jacob's) wicked cleverness, while another part was filled with horror at the things being done.

It was also interesting to note that Jacob was described as a grossly obese man who yielded to all the temptations of the flesh, but predominantly to over-eating rich foods and drinking of a lot of strong beer. During the regression Alison described to me her 'fat white hands', her 'huge paunch' and her 'several chins'.

When the session was over and we were discussing what had occurred, Alison expressed her revulsion at

Jacob's character and her initial distress to think that she could ever have been anyone so horrible in a previous life. I explained to her that today's person bears no responsibility for the way that he or she might have behaved in a previous incarnation and that, indeed, we must all have been either foolish or wicked at some time or we would surely have progressed by now to a state of evolution where we no longer needed to live as human beings.

Suppose that what Alison underwent was an actual regression to a previous life. Because of her experience as Jacob, it is not difficult to see what must have been the link in Alison's mind between gross obesity and evil. Of course she had taken it a stage further and had become obsessive about being thin (as opposed to slim), as if to ensure that there was no way in which she could ever do physical harm to anyone.

Now let us assume that there is no such thing as reincarnation and that Alison's experience had been a mere flight of fancy – an attempt by her subconscious mind to find an explanation for her desperate desire to weigh as little as possible. The effect would be precisely the same.

Whatever the truth of the matter, somewhere deep in Alison's subconscious was the feeling that, should she ever allow herself to become overweight, she would at the same time develop evil tendencies – even though she might not actually go as far as murdering anyone. For this reason, although as a small child she had quite enjoyed her food, as she grew older she could not bear to see her body growing larger. Alison's own belief was that she had experienced an actual reincarnation. Indeed, I think that this belief actually helped with her treatment as she was able to put the blame for her problem on someone else – even if that someone else was a former 'self'.

Follow-up treatment: second consultation
The next time I saw Alison I hypnotized her and asked her to visualize herself standing on one side of a solid brick wall. On the other side of this wall, and quite unable

to see or have any contact with her, was Jacob. I asked her to describe both of these images to me from a purely visual standpoint – nothing whatsoever to do with character or personality. She was able to do this quite easily with Jacob, but when it came to her own image she still saw herself as being far plumper than she really was. I brought her out of the hypnotic state and asked her to measure her bust, waist and hips (which of course were far below average for her height). I then hypnotized her again and asked her to describe herself once more. On this occasion she was able to see herself as (in her words) 'very slim' – she did not actually say 'too thin'. Her homework over the next two weeks was to repeat this image daily, combining it as ever with a relaxation session.

Follow-up treatment: third consultation
When I saw her two weeks later, Alison had a far more realistic view of herself and her size. On this occasion we concentrated on talking about the regression and the reason for her fear of becoming fat. I also hypnotized her again and helped her to visualize Jacob receding further and further into the background, while her own image remained clear.

Cured
After that I saw Alison fortnightly, giving her support through hypnosis and counselling while she learnt to eat normally again. On each occasion we also spent some time talking about Jacob and relegating him to where he belonged – firmly in the past where he could have no further influence on the present-day life of my patient.

Now it might seem wrong to base a cure on treatment which involved the shedding of responsibility for the initial problem, but once again I would suggest that, as long as the cure takes place, it does not really matter. In this case, because Alison could now see a reason for her obsession with thinness, she no longer needed the obsession itself. Of course I am over-simplifying the situation, and her course of treatment involved more than simply identifying the basic cause of the problem; but none the less without that identification all the treatment in the world would have had little (or at best temporary) effect. As it was, by the end of our final consultation, some three months later, Alison was already beginning to eat normally and to put on weight. I had no doubt that, although she would probably never be fat, she would go on to reach an average weight for her age and height.

Although regression therapy and subsequent treatment worked exceptionally well for Alison, none of it would have been possible without initial close liaison with the doctors and specialists who had examined her and found that she was not suffering from anorexia nervosa, as had initially been believed, nor was there any physiological cause for her inability to put on weight. This is why it is imperative that, before embarking on a course of regression therapy for any problem which causes physical symptoms, as many avenues as possible should be explored to ensure that there is no obvious medical reason for the situation.

Sense of inferiority

Roland did not suffer from physical symptoms at all. His condition was psychologically based – but caused him no less distress for all that. On his first visit he crept timidly – almost apologetically – into my consulting room and sat in the chair, eyes downcast and fingers twisting together nervously. It was some time before he could even bring himself to give me details of his name and address, let alone tell me what was troubling him. Eventually he looked at me out of tear-filled eyes and told me that life was just not worth living.

After further gentle questioning on my part, Roland said that he considered himself a weak and useless individual, put upon and treated with contempt by all with whom he came into contact. He had worked for a large company for fifteen years and had seen all those who joined at the same time as he had being promoted not just once but several times, while he remained in the same comparatively lowly position he had occupied for the last twelve of those fifteen years.

He was now by far the oldest in his department and believed that he was looked upon with amusement and contempt by his younger colleagues. His department head was barely civil to him and treated him almost like an office boy, although Roland was in fact both conscientious and capable. However, he was in such terror of losing his job and being unable to find another that he was quite unable to say 'no' when anything was asked of him. As a result it was always Roland who was given the most unpopular tasks, Roland who had to stay late when an emergency arose and Roland who was asked to do so many 'little extras' that he often needed to come into the office on Saturday mornings or had to take work home with him.

As if this were not enough of a problem, matters at home were even worse. His wife, Jean, and their three teenage children treated him with as little respect as his colleagues at work. This situation had been going on for years; indeed Roland could not remember it being any different. His wife had always been a dominant and forceful personality, and he had fallen in with her wishes rather than cause a scene. He had never been able to cope with raised voices or abusive language – something which had caused him to be repeatedly bullied while at school.

Throughout the marriage it had always been Jean who had made the decisions affecting their lifestyle. She decided where they should live, what they should spend and where they should take their holidays. When the babies were born, it was Jean who took complete control of them, scarcely allowing Roland to touch them. As they grew older, it was always their mother they would run to for comfort or advice, and it did not take them long to adopt her contemptuous attitude towards their father.

While fully understanding that no man in his late forties can lightly contemplate throwing away a regular job, however unhappy he may be, many might wonder why Roland remained in what was so obviously a distressing marriage. But, you see, this man had such a low opinion of himself and his worth that he almost agreed that his wife and children were right to treat him as they did. Where a more confident man would never allow such a situation to continue – indeed, probably would not have allowed it to arise in the first place – Roland could not see the possibility of any alternative. Here was a man who was almost happy to be unhappy.

And yet, somewhere beneath all that timidity and self-dislike there must have been a spark of strength and determination, or he would never have come to consult me in the first place. It was this knowledge that made me hope that Roland could indeed be helped.

Beginning the treatment
The first thing to do was to try and establish how long this situation had been going on; I asked Roland to think back and see if he could remember a time when he had been more sure of himself and more assertive. Alas, he could not think of a single occasion. Even as a small child he had lived in fear of his two older and more outgoing brothers; and, because he had been intimidated by their threats of physical violence, they had been able to force him to carry out their household chores for them. He did not know whether his parents were unaware of the situation or whether they simply did nothing about it. In any event, his brothers were never chastised for their attitude, so that eventually they did not even bother to hide it. However, this did not seem to me to be sufficient grounds for his present self-image and I felt that it might be beneficial to explore further.

Having explained to him about regression, and with his complete acquiescence, I hypnotized Roland and tried taking him back to very early stages in this lifetime. All that he had consciously remembered appeared to be true. There did not seem to be a single occasion when he was aware of having been a positive and assertive individual.

113

Looking at past lives

I decided therefore to regress him to a previous life and see if we could discover what could possibly have given him his abnormally low opinion of himself. Roland was a little nervous, but had by now become so desperate to find some cause for his attitude that he was willing to try almost anything.

Because of his nervousness he was not an easy person to regress. Although we had worked together on the relaxation part of the hypnotic state, on this occasion he found it extremely difficult. It was almost as though he did not want to discover the initial cause of his problem. This is not altogether unusual: even when someone is in an unhappy position, they have often become so used to it that to remove it is like taking away their security blanket; they are terrified of being left in a vacuum with no personality at all. Because of this I reassured Roland that, whatever we discovered during the course of the regression, in later sessions we would work towards the building of a new and stronger persona so that he need have no fear about being left to flounder in a sea of nothingness.

Once he had relaxed sufficiently for the session of past-life regression to take place, Roland quickly reached a stage where he was able to tell me about a former life. He described to me a life of misery as a slave to a band of travelling people in seventeenth-century Europe. Apparently he had been taken from his family by these people when he was just a baby, for he could remember no other life. He knew, however, that he was not one of them. His skin was pale whereas their's was swarthy; his hair was fair and his eyes blue, while they were dark-eyed and had hair as black as a raven's wing. As their slave he had to perform the most menial and unsavoury tasks but, although he felt hatred and animosity towards them, he had been so badly abused and so humiliated that he did not dare to express it.

I was intrigued to note that, even during such a miserable existence, Roland was at least able to feel anger and

114

hatred towards his captors – this was something he did not feel capable of evoking during his twentieth-century life, tending instead to put up with what others said and did and even to justify their words and actions by expressing his own low opinion of himself. In that earlier life, however, although he did not dare to demonstrate his anger in any way for fear of physical repercussions, none the less the emotion was present – and this I felt would be of positive help to Roland when we went on to deal with his current problem.

The session of past-life regression was not a long one, as the poor slave suffered such a deprived and pitiful life that he died before reaching full maturity. Because of the detachment technique described earlier (see p.26), the incidence of death itself is not distressing for the person undergoing that regression even when the life itself has been a happy one. In Roland's case the existence had been so miserable that he was quite happy to lay down the yoke of life when the time came.

Now it is possible – indeed, I think it is probable – that Roland actually did re-experience a former existence of his own. If he did, and if all that he related was true, one could easily see why he had brought with him the inner belief that he was worth less than those around him and that he must therefore put up with their contempt and their low opinion of him. As we have already seen, it is possible that the spirit has to learn to cope with a series of different lessons as it makes its journey towards complete evolvement; if success is not achieved during one lifetime, the spirit will be faced with it again and again during the course of future lives until the lesson has finally been learnt.

Suppose, however, that what Roland experienced was not really a glimpse into a past life but simply a desperate attempt on the part of his subconscious mind to make excuses for his lack of assertiveness and his poor self-image during his present life. Once again, does it really matter? As you will see below when we come to deal with the follow-up treatment involved in this case, the results would be precisely the same.

At the end of that particular session I actually asked Roland whether he felt that he had truly remembered events which had happened to him in a former life or whether he believed that it was his imagination playing tricks and conjuring up a plausible story. He had no doubt in his mind, because of the vividness of what he had experienced, that he had indeed recalled a miserable but significant previous existence.

Follow-up treatment

When working with a patient who has a poor self-image and is therefore devoid of confidence, the process is quite slow. If only there were some way of hypnotizing him and saying, 'You will now be confident' – but it just does not work like that. We have to start with one very small area where the patient would like to be more sure of himself (or herself). In Roland's case he wanted to be able to say 'no' at work when the need arose. He had no intention of being aggressive or belligerent – indeed, this would not have been possible. He simply felt that he no longer wished to be put upon and to be the one who always ended up staying late or doing the jobs that no one else wanted to do.

Having hypnotized him, I asked Roland to visualize a typical situation where this problem might arise. He imagined his department manager asking him to stay after work and do some filing, even though he had arranged to go the cinema with his wife that evening. To have suggested to Roland that he should say a flat 'No, I won't' would have been ridiculous; for one thing, he would have been incapable of doing so, and for another, I did not want to be responsible for causing friction between him and his boss. So Roland imagined himself being very calm and pleasant and explaining to the manager about his pre-arranged outing and the reason why he could not stay in the office. His homework was to continue using this image until he felt quite comfortable with it and was able to react in this way at work.

From there we went on – one step at a time – to deal in a similar way with other areas of Roland's life which bothered him and where he felt capable of changing. The process was a fairly slow one, as it is important that we always work at the patient's own pace and poor Roland had a lifetime of timidity behind him. He would never become a loud and assertive personality – but he had no desire to do so. He simply wanted to think better of himself and to deal with the situations which had caused him the most distress.

Roland was a patient of mine for about four months, by the end of which time he felt that he had improved considerably. Perhaps the most important point was that he felt better about himself. After that I saw him two or three times a year (and I still do), whenever he feels that things are getting on top of him again.

Conclusion

Regression, when properly controlled and guided, can achieve so much. Whether we are dealing with deeply traumatic problems in the past or a desire to improve one's talent in the future, it is one of the most positive tools in the hypnotherapist's workbox. We are all influenced far more than we realize by things which were said or done, events which happened, or people with whom we have been in contact in the past - whether we remember them or not. Since there is in existence a therapy which allows us to make use of those memories, however deeply hidden they may be, it seems only sensible to take advantage of that therapy in order to create for ourselves a happier and more fulfilling life in the future.

Bibliography

French, Neil, *Successful Hypnotherapy* (Thorsons, 1984)
Goldberg, Dr Bruce, *Past Lives, Future Lives* (Newcastle Publishing Co., 1982)
Markham, Ursula, *Hypnosis* (Optima, 1987)
Moody, Raymond A., and Paul Perry, *Life Before Life* (Macmillan, 1990)
Roet, Dr Brian, *Hypnosis - A Gateway to Better Health* (Weidenfeld & Nicolson, 1986)
Wambach, Helen, *Reliving Past Lives* (Hutchinson, 1979)

Cassettes

There are a few cassettes on the market which claim to assist the listener to experience regression on his own. Because of my conviction that no one should ever undergo any form of regression unless in the presence of an experienced therapist, I would suggest that such cassettes should be avoided. Cassettes which are designed to help the listener become accustomed to hypnotherapy and the relaxation which is an integral part of it can, however, prove extremely useful. Such cassettes are available from:

Thorsons Publishing Group Ltd
78–85 Fulham Palace Road
London
W6 8JB

The Hypnothink Foundation
PO Box 154
Cheltenham
Gloucestershire
GL53 9EG

Addresses

The following organizations will be able to give information about members practising regression therapy. (A stamped addressed envelope will be appreciated.)

Great Britain

British Society of Hypnotherapy
37 Orbain Road
London
SW6 7JZ

International Association of Hypnoanalysts
The Hypnotherapy Centre
PO Box 180
1, Lowther Gardens
Bournemouth
Dorset
BH8 8NH

World Federation of Hypnotherapists
46 Belmont Road
Ramsgate
Kent
CT11 7QG

The Hypnothink Foundation
PO Box 154
Cheltenham
Gloucestershire
GL53 9EG

Ireland

Irish Society for Clinical and Experimental Hypnosis
49 McCurtain Street
Cork
Eire

Australia

Australian Society of Hypnosis
PO Box 366
Glenleg
S. Australia 5045

New Zealand

Erna Moss
33 Duncansby Road
Whangaporoa 12167

Canada

Ontario Society for Clinical Hypnosis
170 St George Street, Ste. 1001
Toronto
Ontario

USA

Association for Past-Life Research and Therapy
PO Box 20151
Riverside
Ca. 92516

Index